Praise for

TERRY TEMPEST WILLIAMS's
Refuge

"This is a book of life and loss and love, harrowing in some parts, heart-warming in others, written in a spare prose that seems to reverberate." —*Seattle Post-Intelligencer*

"The courage, the passion, and the purity of motive in Terry Tempest Williams's voice are remarkable. Her demonstration of how deeply human emotional life can become intertwined with a particular landscape could not be more relevant to our lives." —Barry Lopez, author of *Arctic Dreams*

"Terry Tempest Williams's honesty is downright searing— searing, and perhaps healing...[She is] a fine writer, and a brave one." —*Wilderness*

"*Refuge* is an intensely private love story of a woman and her landscape—the one she sees with her eyes and the one mirrored by her heart." —*Salt Lake Tribune*

"Williams is a remarkable writer....This book is more than a pleasure to read, it offers a disturbing message for all to consider. I found myself ruminating on it long after I had closed the cover for the final time." —*Jackson Hole News*

"*Refuge* is an almost unbearably intense and skillful essay on mortality, our own and that of the creative world. It is isolated from nearly all others of the genre by Ms. Williams's 'greatness of soul'—there is no other way to express the dense beauty and grace of this book." —Jim Harrison, author of *Legends of the Fall*

"*Refuge* is a simultaneously courageous and graceful book." —*Durango Herald*

"The wonderful thing about *Refuge* is that Terry Williams is too full of life herself, and too fascinated by all its manifestations, to write a gloomy book. There isn't a page in *Refuge* that doesn't whistle with the sound of wings." —Wallace Stegner

BY THE SAME AUTHOR

The Secret Language of Snow (with Ted Major)

Pieces of White Shell: A Journey to Navajoland

Between Cattails

Coyote's Canyon

Earthly Messengers

An Unspoken Hunger

Desert Quartet

TERRY TEMPEST WILLIAMS
Refuge

Terry Tempest Williams is Naturalist-in-Residence at the Utah Museum of Natural History in Salt Lake City. Her first book, *Pieces of White Shell: A Journey to Navajoland* (1984), received the 1984 Southwest Book Award. She is also the author of *Coyote's Canyon* and of two children's books. Terry Tempest Williams lives in Salt Lake City.

For you John
In the name of
the Spirit that moves us,
and heals

REFUGE

*An Unnatural
History of Family and Place*

Fondly,

Terry Tempest Williams

Terry Tempest Williams

*6 October 98
SLC*

Vintage Books
A Division of Random House, Inc.
New York

FIRST VINTAGE BOOKS EDITION, SEPTEMBER 1992

"The Clan of One-Breasted Women" by Terry Tempest Williams was originally published in Northern Lights, January 1990, Volume VI, No. 1.

Grateful acknowledgment is made to the following for permission to reprint previously published material: Atlantic Monthly Press: "Wild Geese" from Dream Work by Mary Oliver. Copyright © 1986 by Mary Oliver. Reprinted by permission of Atlantic Monthly Press.

Harcourt Brace Jovanovich, Inc.: "The Peace of Wild Things" from Openings by Wendell Berry. Reprinted by permission of Harcourt Brace Jovanovich, Inc.

Library of Congress Cataloging-in-Publication Data

Williams, Terry Tempest.
    Refuge / Terry Tempest Williams. — 1st Vintage ed.
      p. cm.
    Originally published: New York: Pantheon Books, © 1991.
    ISBN 0-679-74024-4 (pbk.)
    1. Williams, Terry Tempest—Health. 2. Breast—Cancer—
    Patients—Utah—Biography. 3. Natural history—Utah—
    Great Salt Lake Region.
  I. Title.
  [RC280.B8W47 1992]
  362.1'9699449'0092—dc20
  [B]   92-50102
          CIP

Book and map design by Anne Scatto

Manufactured in the United States of America

For
Diane Dixon Tempest
who understood landscape as refuge

WILD GEESE

You do not have to be good.
You do not have to walk on your knees
for a hundred miles through the desert, repenting.
You only have to let the soft animal of your body love
  what it loves.
Tell me about despair, yours, and I will tell you mine.
Meanwhile the world goes on.
Meanwhile the sun and the clear pebbles of the rain
are moving across the landscapes,
over the prairies and deep trees,
the mountains and the rivers.
Meanwhile the wild geese, high in the clean blue air
are heading home again.
Whoever you are, no matter how lonely,
the world offers itself to your imagination,
calls to you like the wild geese, harsh and exciting—
over and over announcing your place
in the family of things.

                    —MARY OLIVER,
                      Dream Work

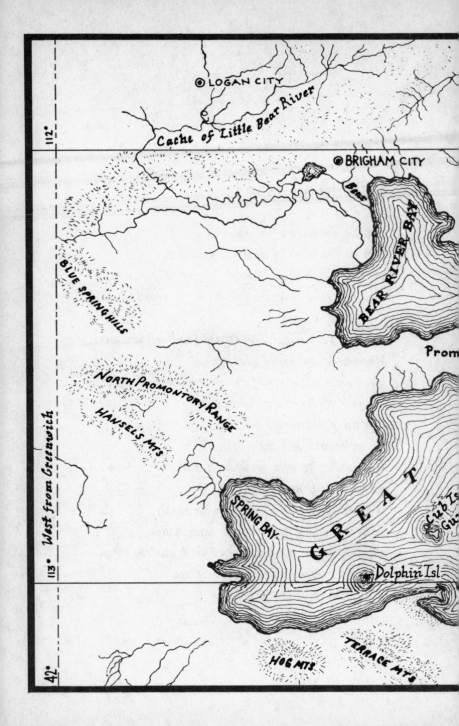

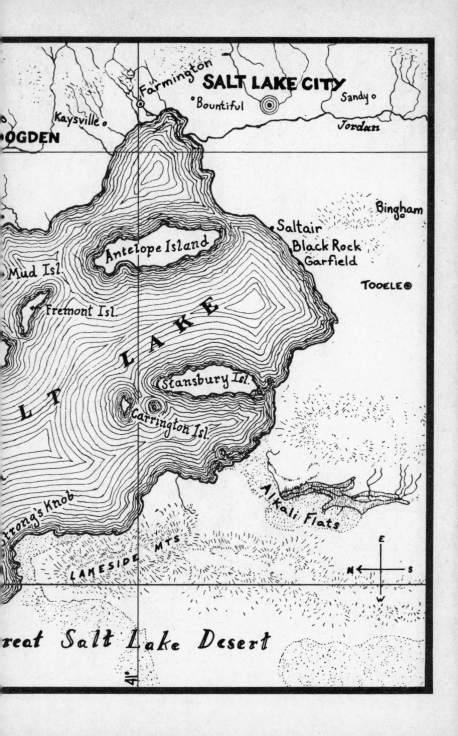

CONTENTS

xiii

Contents

Contents

REFUGE

PROLOGUE

Everything about Great Salt Lake is exaggerated—the heat, the cold, the salt, and the brine. It is a landscape so surreal one can never know what it is for certain.

In the past seven years, Great Salt Lake has advanced and retreated. The Bear River Migratory Bird Refuge, devastated by the flood, now begins to heal. Volunteers are beginning to reconstruct the marshes just as I am trying to reconstruct my life. I sit on the floor of my study with journals all around me. I open them and feathers fall from their pages, sand cracks their spines, and sprigs of sage pressed between passages of pain heighten my sense of smell—and I remember the country I come from and how it informs my life.

Most of the women in my family are dead. Cancer. At thirty-four, I became the matriarch of my family. The losses I encountered at the Bear River Migratory Bird Refuge as

Great Salt Lake was rising helped me to face the losses within my family. When most people had given up on the Refuge, saying the birds were gone, I was drawn further into its essence. In the same way that when someone is dying many retreat, I chose to stay.

Last night, I dreamed I was walking along the shores of Great Salt Lake. I noticed a purple bird floating in the waters, the waves rocking it gently. I entered the lake and, with cupped hands, picked up the bird and returned it to shore. The purple bird turned gold, dropped its tail, and began digging a burrow in the white sand, where it retreated and sealed itself inside with salt. I walked away. It was dusk. The next day, I returned to the lake shore. A wooden door frame, freestanding, became an arch I had to walk through. Suddenly, it was transformed into Athene's Temple. The bird was gone. I was left standing with my own memory.

In the next segment of the dream, I was in a doctor's office. He said, "You have cancer in your blood and you have nine months to heal yourself." I awoke puzzled and frightened.

Perhaps, I am telling this story in an attempt to heal myself, to confront what I do not know, to create a path for myself with the idea that "memory is the only way home."

I have been in retreat. This story is my return.

TTW
JULY 4, 1990

BURROWING OWLS

lake level: 4204.70'

Great Salt Lake is about twenty-five minutes from our home. From the mouth of Emigration Canyon where we live, I drive west past Brigham Young standing on top of "This Is the Place" monument. When I reach Foothill Drive, I turn right, pass the University of Utah and make another right, heading east until I meet South Temple, which requires a left-hand turn. I arrive a few miles later at Eagle Gate, a bronze arch that spans State Street. I turn right once more. One block later, I turn left on North Temple and pass the Mormon Tabernacle on Temple Square. From here, I simply follow the gulls west, past the Salt Lake City International Airport.

Great Salt Lake: wilderness adjacent to a city; a shifting shoreline that plays havoc with highways; islands too stark, too remote to inhabit; water in the desert that no one can drink. It is the liquid lie of the West.

I recall an experiment from school: we filled a cup with water—the surface area of the contents was only a few square inches. Then we poured the same amount of water into a large, shallow dinner plate—it covered nearly a square foot. Most lakes in the world are like cups of water. Great Salt Lake, with its average depth measuring only thirteen feet, is like the dinner plate. We then added two or three tablespoons of salt to the cup of water for the right amount of salinity to complete the analogue.

The experiment continued: we let the plate and cup of water stand side by side on the window sill. As they evaporated, we watched the plate of water dry up becoming encrusted with salt long before the cup. The crystals were beautiful.

Because Great Salt Lake lies on the bottom of the Great Basin, the largest closed system in North America, it is a terminal lake with no outlet to the sea.

The water level of Great Salt Lake fluctuates wildly in response to climatic changes. The sun bears down on the lake an average of about 70 percent of the time. The water frequently reaches ninety degrees Fahrenheit, absorbing enough energy to evaporate almost four feet of water annually. If rainfall exceeds the evaporation rate, Great Salt Lake rises. If rainfall drops below the evaporation rate, the lake recedes. Add the enormous volume of stream inflow from the high Wasatch and Uinta Mountains in the east, and one begins to see a portrait of change.

Great Salt Lake is cyclic. At winter's end, the lake level rises with mountain runoff. By late spring, it begins to decline when the weather becomes hot enough that loss of water by evaporation from the surface is greater than the combined inflow from streams, ground water, and precipitation. The lake begins to rise again in the autumn, when the temperature decreases, and the loss of water by evaporation is exceeded by the inflow.

Since Captain Howard Stansbury's *Exploration and Survey of the Great Salt Lake, 1852,* the water level has varied by as much as twenty feet, altering the shoreline in some places by as much as fifteen miles. Great Salt Lake is surrounded by salt flats, sage plains, and farmland; a slight rise in the water level extends its area considerably. In the past twenty years, Great Salt Lake's surface area has fluctuated from fifteen hundred square miles to its present twenty-five hundred square miles. Great Salt Lake is now approximately the size of Delaware and Rhode Island. It has been estimated that a ten foot rise in Great Salt Lake would cover an additional two hundred forty square miles.

To understand the relationship that exists at Great Salt Lake between area and volume, imagine pouring one inch of water into the bottom of a paper cone. It doesn't take much water to raise an inch. However, if you wanted to raise the water level one inch at the top of the cone, the volume of water added would have to increase considerably. The lake bed of Great Salt Lake is cone-shaped. It takes more water to raise the lake an inch when it is at high-level, and less water to raise it in low-level years.

Natives of the Great Basin, of the Salt Lake Valley in particular, speak about Great Salt Lake in the shorthand of lake levels. For example, in 1963, Great Salt Lake retreated to its historic low of 4191'. Ten years later, Great Salt Lake reached its historic mean, 4200'—about the same level explorers John Fremont and Howard Stansbury encountered in the 1840s and 50s.

On September 18, 1982, Great Salt Lake began to rise because of a series of storms that occurred earlier in the month. The precipitation of 7.04 inches for the month (compared to an annual average of about fifteen inches from 1875 to 1982) made it the wettest September on record for Salt Lake City. The lake continued to rise for the next ten months as a result of greater-than-average snowfall during the winter and spring of 1982–83, and unseasonably cool weather (thus little evaporation) during the spring of 1983. The rise from September 18, 1982 to June 30, 1983, was 5.1', the greatest seasonal rise ever recorded.

During these years, talk on the streets of Salt Lake City has centered around the lake: 4204' and rising. It is no longer just a backdrop for spectacular sunsets. It is the play of urban drama. Everyone has their interests. 4211.6' was the historic high recorded in the 1870's. City officials knew the Salt Lake City International Airport would be underwater if the Great Salt Lake rose to 4220'. Developments along the lakeshore were sunk at 4208'. Farmers whose land was being flooded in daily increments were trying desperately to dike or sell. And the Southern Pacific Railroad labors to maintain their tracks above water, twenty-four hours a day, three hundred sixty-five days a year, and has been doing so since 1959.

My interest lay at 4206', the level which, according to my topographical map, meant the flooding of the Bear River Migratory Bird Refuge.

There are those birds you gauge your life by. The burrowing owls five miles from the entrance to the Bear River Migratory Bird Refuge are mine. Sentries. Each year, they alert me to the regularities of the land. In spring, I find them nesting, in summer they forage with their young, and by winter they abandon the Refuge for a place more comfortable.

What is distinctive about these owls is their home. It rises from the alkaline flats like a clay-covered fist. If you were to peek inside the tightly clenched fingers, you would find a dark-holed entrance.

"Tttss! Tttss! Tttss!"

That is no rattlesnake. Those are the distress cries of the burrowing owl's young.

Adult burrowing owls will stand on top of the mound with their prey before them, usually small rodents, birds, or insects. The entrance is littered with bones and feathers. I recall finding a swatch of yellow feathers like a doormat across the threshold—meadowlark, maybe. These small owls pursue their prey religiously at dusk.

Burrowing owls are part of the desert community, taking advantage of the abandoned burrows of prairie dogs. Historically, bison would move across the American Plains, followed by prairie dog towns which would aerate the soil after the weight of stampeding hooves. Black-footed ferrets, rattlesnakes, and burrowing owls inhabited the edges, finding an abundant food source in the communal rodents.

With the loss of desert lands, a decline in prairie dog populations is inevitable. And so go the ferret and burrowing owl. Rattlesnakes are more adaptable.

In Utah, prairie dogs and black-footed ferrets are endangered species, with ferrets almost extinct. The burrowing owl is defined as "threatened," a political step away from endangered status. Each year, the burrowing owls near the Refuge become more blessed.

The owls had staked their territory just beyond one of the bends in the Bear River. Whenever I drove to the Bird Refuge, I stopped at their place first and sat on the edge of the road and watched. They would fly around me, their wings sometimes spanning two feet. Undulating from post to post, they would distract me from their nest. Just under a foot long, they have a body of feathers the color of wheat, balanced on two long, spindly legs. They can burn grasses with their stare. Yellow eyes magnifying light.

The protective hissing of baby burrowing owls is an adaptive memory of their close association with prairie rattlers. Snake or owl? Who wants to risk finding out.

In the summer of 1983, I worried about the burrowing owls, wondering if the rising waters of Great Salt Lake had flooded their home, too. I was relieved to find not only their mound intact, but four owlets standing on its threshold. One of the Refuge managers stopped on the road and commented on what a good year it had been for them.

"Good news," I replied. "The lake didn't take everything."

That was late August when huge concentrations of shorebirds were still feeding between submerged shadescale.

A few months later, a friend of mine, Sandy Lopez, was visiting from Oregon. We had spoken of the Bird Refuge many times. The whistling swans had arrived, and it seemed like a perfect day for the marsh.

To drive to the Bear River Migratory Bird Refuge from Salt Lake City takes a little over one hour. I have discovered the conversation that finds its way into the car often manifests itself later on the land.

We spoke of rage. Of women and landscape. How our bodies and the body of the earth have been mined.

"It has everything to do with intimacy," I said. "Men define intimacy through their bodies. It is physical. They define intimacy with the land in the same way."

"Many men have forgotten what they are connected to," my friend added. "Subjugation of women and nature may be a loss of intimacy within themselves."

She paused, then looked at me.

"Do you feel rage?"

I didn't answer for some time.

"I feel sadness. I feel powerless at times. But I'm not certain what rage really means."

Several miles passed.

"Do you?" I asked.

She looked out the window. "Yes. Perhaps your generation, one behind mine, is a step removed from the pain."

We reached the access road to the Refuge and both took out our binoculars, ready for the birds. Most of the waterfowl had migrated, but a few ruddy ducks, redheads, and shovelers remained. The marsh glistened like cut topaz.

As we turned west about five miles from the Refuge, a mile or so from the burrowing owl's mound, I began to speak of them, *Athene cunicularia*. I told Sandy about the time when my grandmother and I first discovered them. It was in 1960, the same year she gave me my Peterson's *Field Guide to Western Birds*. I know because I dated their picture. We have come back every year since to pay our respects. Generations of burrowing owls have been raised here. I turned to my friend and explained how four owlets had survived the flood.

We anticipated them.

About a half mile away, I could not see the mound. I took my foot off the gas pedal and coasted. It was as though I was in unfamiliar country.

The mound was gone. Erased. In its place, fifty feet back, stood a cinderblock building with a sign, CANADIAN GOOSE GUN CLUB. A new fence crushed the grasses with a handwritten note posted: KEEP OUT.

We got out of the car and walked to where the mound had been for as long as I had a memory. Gone. Not a pellet to be found.

A blue pickup pulled alongside us.

"Howdy." They tipped their ball caps. "What y'all loo-kin' for?"

I said nothing. Sandy said nothing. My eyes narrowed.

"We didn't kill 'em. Those boys from the highway de-partment came and graveled the place. Two bits, they did it. I mean, you gotta admit those ground owls are messy little bastards. They'll shit all over hell if ya let 'em. And try and sleep with 'em hollering at ya all night long. They had to go. Anyway, we got bets with the county they'll pop up someplace around here next year."

The three men in the front seat looked up at us, tipped their caps again. And drove off.

Restraint is the steel partition between a rational mind and a violent one. I knew rage. It was fire in my stomach with no place to go.

I drove out to the Refuge on another day. I suppose I wanted to see the mound back in place with the family of owls bobbing on top. Of course, they were not.

I sat on the gravel and threw stones.

By chance, the same blue pickup with the same three men pulled alongside: the self-appointed proprietors of the newly erected Canadian Goose Gun Club.

"Howdy, ma'am. Still lookin' for them owls, or was it sparrows?"

One winked.

Suddenly in perfect detail, I pictured the burrowing owls' mound—that clay-covered fist rising from the alkaline flats. The exact one these beergut-over-beltbuckled men had lev-eled.

I walked calmly over to their truck and leaned my stom-ach against their door. I held up my fist a few inches from the driver's face and slowly lifted my middle finger to the sky.

"This is for you—from the owls and me."

My mother was appalled—not so much over the loss of the burrowing owls, although it saddened her, but by my behavior. Women did not deliver obscene gestures to men, regardless. She shook her head, saying she had no idea where I came from.

In Mormon culture, that is one of the things you do know—history and geneology. I come from a family with deep roots in the American West. When the expense of outfitting several thousand immigrants to Utah was becoming too great for the newly established church, leaders decided to furnish the pioneers with small two-wheeled carts about the size of those used by apple peddlers, which could be pulled by hand from Missouri to the Salt Lake Valley. My ancestors were part of these original "handcart companies" in the 1850s. With faith, they would endure. They came with few provisions over the twelve-hundred-mile trail. It was a small sacrifice in the name of religious freedom. Almost one hundred and fifty years later, we are still here.

I am the oldest child in our family, a daughter with three younger brothers: Steve, Dan, and Hank.

My parents, John Henry Tempest, III, and Diane Dixon Tempest, were married in the Mormon Temple in Salt Lake City on September 18, 1953. My husband, Brooke Williams, and I followed the same tradition and were married on June 2, 1975. I was nineteen years old.

Our extended family includes both maternal and paternal grandparents: Lettie Romney Dixon and Donald "Sanky" Dixon, Kathryn Blackett Tempest and John Henry Tempest, Jr.

Aunts, uncles, and cousins are many, extending familial ties all across the state of Utah. If I ever wonder who I am, I simply attend a Romney family reunion and find myself in the eyes of everyone I meet. It is comforting and disturbing, at once.

I have known five of my great-grandparents intimately. They tutored me in stories with a belief that lineage mattered. Genealogy is in our blood. As a people and as a family, we have a sense of history. And our history is tied to land.

I was raised to believe in a spirit world, that life exists before the earth and will continue to exist afterward, that each human being, bird, and bulrush, along with all other life forms had a spirit life before it came to dwell physically on the earth. Each occupied an assigned sphere of influence, each has a place and a purpose.

It made sense to a child. And if the natural world was assigned spiritual values, then those days spent in wildness were sacred. We learned at an early age that God can be found wherever you are, especially outside. Family worship was not just relegated to Sunday in a chapel.

Our weekends were spent camped alongside a small stream in the Great Basin, in the Stansbury Mountains or Deep Creeks. My father would take the boys rabbit hunting while Mother and I would sit on a log in an aspen grove and talk. She would tell me stories of how when she was a girl she would paint red lips on the trunks of trees to practice kissing. Or how she would lie in her grandmother's lucerne patch and watch clouds.

"I have never known my full capacity for solitude," she would say.

"Solitude?" I asked.

"The gift of being alone. I can never get enough."

The men would return anxious for dinner. Mother would cook over a green Coleman stove as Dad told stories from his childhood—like the time his father took away his BB gun for a year because he shot off the heads of every red tulip in his mother's garden, row after row after row. He laughed. We laughed. And then it was time to bless the food.

After supper, we would spread out our sleeping bags in a circle, heads pointing to the center like a covey of quail, and watch the Great Basin sky fill with stars. Our attachment to the land was our attachment to each other.

The days I loved most were the days at Bear River. The Bird Refuge was a sanctuary for my grandmother and me. I call her "Mimi." We would walk along the road with binoculars around our necks and simply watch birds. Hundreds of birds. Birds so exotic to a desert child it forced the imagination to be still. The imagined was real at Bear River.

I recall one bird in particular. It wore a feathered robe of cinnamon, white, and black. Its body rested on long, thin legs. Blue legs. On the edge of the marsh, it gracefully lowered its head and began sweeping the water side to side with its delicate, upturned bill.

"Plee-ek! Plee-ek! Plee-ek!"

Three more landed. My grandmother placed her hand gently on my shoulder and whispered, "avocets." I was nine years old.

At ten, Mimi thought I was old enough to join the

Audubon Society on a special outing to the wetlands surrounding Great Salt Lake. We boarded a greyhound bus in downtown Salt Lake and drove north on U.S. Highway 91, paralleling the Wasatch Mountains on our right and Great Salt Lake on our left. Once relaxed and out of the city, we were handed an official checklist of birds at the Bear River Migratory Bird Refuge.

"All members are encouraged to take copious notes and keep scrupulous records of birds seen," proclaimed the gray-haired, ponytailed woman passing out cards.

"What do copious and scrupulous mean?" I asked my grandmother.

"It means pay attention," she said. I pulled out my notebook and drew pictures of the backs of birdwatchers' heads.

Off the highway, the bus drove through the small town of Brigham City with its sycamore-lined streets. It's like most Utah settlements with its Mormon layout: a chapel for weekly worship, a tabernacle for communal events, and a temple nearby (in this case Logan) where sacred rites are performed. Lawns are well groomed and neighborhoods are immaculate. But the banner arched over Main Street makes this town unique. In neon lights it reads, BRIGHAM CITY: GATEWAY TO THE WORLD'S GREATEST GAME BIRD REFUGE. So welded to the local color of this community, I daresay no one sees the sign anymore, except newcomers and perhaps the birds that fly under it.

A small, elderly man with wire-rimmed glasses and a worn golf cap, stood at the front of the bus and began speaking into the handheld microphone: "Ladies and gentlemen, in approximately ten miles we will be entering the Bear River Migratory Bird Refuge, America's first waterfowl sanctuary, established by a special act of Congress on April 23, 1928."

I was confused. I thought the marsh had been created in

the spirit world first and on earth second. I never made the connection that God and Congress were in cahoots. Mimi said she would explain the situation later.

The man went on to say that the Bird Refuge was located at the delta of the Bear River, which poured into the Great Salt Lake. This I understood.

"People, this bus is a clock. Eyes forward, please. Straight ahead is twelve o'clock; to the rear is six. Three o'clock is on your right. Any bird identified from this point on will be noted accordingly."

The bus became a bird dog, a labrador on wheels, which decided where high noon would be simply by pointing in that direction. What time would it be if a bird decided to fly from nine o'clock to three o'clock? Did that make the bird half past nine or quarter to three? Even more worrisome to me was the possibility of a flock of birds flying between four and five o'clock. Would you say, "Twenty birds after four? Four-thirty? Or simply move the hands of the clock forward to five? I decided not to bother my grandmother with these particulars and, instead, retreated to my unindexed field guide and turned to the color plates of ducks.

"Ibises at two o'clock!"

The brakes squeaked the bus to a halt. The doors opened like bellows and we all filed out. And there they were, dozens of white-faced glossy ibises grazing in the field. Their feathers on first glance were chestnut, but with the slightest turn they flashed irridescences of pink, purple, and green.

Another flock landed nearby. And another. And another. They coasted in diagonal lines with their heads and necks extended, their long legs trailing behind them, seeming to fall forward on hinges the second before they touched ground. By now, we must have been watching close to a hundred ibises probing the farmlands adjacent to the marsh.

Our leader told us they were eating earthworms and insects.

"Good eyes," I thought, as I could only see their decurved bills like scythes disappearing behind the grasses. I watched the wind turn each feather as the birds turned the soil.

Mimi whispered to me how ibises are the companions of gods. "Ibis escorts Thoth, the Egyptian god of wisdom and magic, who is the guardian of the Moon Gates in heaven. And there are two colors of ibis—one black and one white. The dark bird is believed to be associated with death, the white bird a celebration of birth."

I looked out over the fields of black ibis.

"When an ibis tucks its head underwing to sleep, it resembles a heart. The ibis knows empathy," my grand-mother said. "Remember that, alongside the fact it eats worms."

She also told me that if I could learn a new way to tell time, I could also learn a new way to measure distance.

"The stride of an ibis was a measurement used in building the great temples of the Nile."

I sat down by the rear wheels of the bus and pondered the relationship between an ibis at Bear River and an ibis foraging on the banks of the Nile. In my young mind, it had something to do with the magic of birds, how they bridge cultures and continents with their wings, how they mediate between heaven and earth.

Back on the bus and moving, I wrote in my notebook "one hundred white-faced glossy ibises—companions of the gods."

Mimi was pleased. "We could go home now," she said. "The ibis makes the day."

But there were more birds. Many, many more. Within the next few miles, ducks, geese, and shorebirds were sighted around "the clock." The bus drove past all of them. With my arms out the window, I tried to touch the wings of avocets and stilts. I knew these birds from our private trips to the Refuge. They had become relatives.

As the black-necked stilts flew alongside the silver bus, their long legs trailed behind them like red streamers.

"Ip-ip-ip! Ip-ip-ip!"

Their bills were not flattened and upturned like avocets, but straight as darning needles.

The wind massaged my face. I closed my eyes and sat back in my seat.

Mimi and I got out of the bus and ate our lunch on the riverbank. Two western grebes, ruby-eyed and serpentine, fished, diving at good prospects. They surfaced with silver minnows struggling between sharp mandibles. Violet-green swallows skimmed the water for midges as a snowy egret stood on the edge of the spillway.

With a crab sandwich in one hand and binoculars in the other, Mimi explained why the Bird Refuge had in fact, been created.

"Maybe the best way to understand it," she said, "is to realize the original wetlands were recreated. It was the deterioration of the marshes at Bear River Bay that led to the establishment of a sanctuary."

"How?" I asked.

"The marshes were declining for several reasons: the diversion of water from the Bear River for irrigation, the backing-up of brine from Great Salt Lake during high-water periods, excessive hunting, and a dramatic rise in botulism, a disease known then as 'western duck disease.'

"The creation of the Bear River Migratory Bird Refuge helped to preserve the freshwater character of the marsh. Dikes were built to hold the water from the Bear River to stabilize, manage, and control water levels within the marsh.

This helped to control botulism and at the same time keep out the brine. Meanwhile, the birds flourished."

After lunch, I climbed the observation tower at the Refuge headquarters. Any fear of heights I may have had moving up the endless flights of steel stairs was replaced by the bird's eye view before me. The marsh appeared as a green and blue mosaic where birds remained in a fluid landscape.

In the afternoon, we drove the twenty-two-mile loop around the Refuge. The roads capped the dikes which were bordered by deep channels of water with bulrush and teasel. We saw ruddy ducks (the man sitting behind us called them "blue bills"), shovelers, teals, and wigeons. We watched herons and egrets and rails. Red-wing blackbirds poised on cattails sang with long-billed marsh wrens as muskrats swam inside shadows created by clouds. Large families of Canada geese occupied the open water, while ravens flushed the edges for unprotected nests with eggs.

The marsh reflected health as concentric circles rippled outward from a mallard feeding "bottoms up."

By the end of the day, Mimi and I had marked sixty-seven species on our checklist, many of which I had never seen before. A short-eared owl hovered over the cattails. It was the last bird we saw as we left the Refuge.

I fell asleep on my grandmother's lap. Her strong, square hands resting on my forehead shielded the sun from my eyes. I dreamed of water and cattails and all that is hidden.

When we returned home, my family was seated around the dinner table.

"What did you see?" Mother asked. My father and three brothers looked up.

"Birds . . ." I said as I closed my eyes and stretched my arms like wings.

"Hundreds of birds at the marsh."

WHIMBRELS

lake level: 4203.25'

The Bird Refuge has remained a constant. It is a landscape so familiar to me, there have been times I have felt a species long before I saw it. The long-billed curlews that foraged the grasslands seven miles outside the Refuge were trustworthy. I can count on them year after year. And when six whimbrels joined them—whimbrel entered my mind as an idea. Before I ever saw them mingling with curlews, I recognized them as a new thought in familiar country.

The birds and I share a natural history. It is a matter of rootedness, of living inside a place for so long that the mind and imagination fuse.

Maybe it's the expanse of sky above and water below that soothes my soul. Or maybe it's the anticipation of seeing something new. Whatever the magic of Bear River is—I appreciate this corner of northern Utah, where the numbers of ducks and geese I find resemble those found by early explorers.

Of the 208 species of birds who use the Refuge, sixty-two are known to nest here. Such nesting species include eared, western, and pied-billed grebes, great blue herons, snowy egrets, white-faced ibises, American avocets, black-necked stilts, and Wilson's phalaropes. Also nesting at Bear River are Canada geese, mallards, gadwalls, pintails, green-winged, blue-winged, and cinnamon teals, redheads, and ruddy ducks. It is a fertile community where the hope of each day rides on the backs of migrating birds.

These wetlands, emeralds around Great Salt Lake, provide critical habitat for North American waterfowl and shore-birds, supporting hundreds of thousands, even millions of individuals during spring and autumn migrations. The long-legged birds with their eyes focused down transform a seemingly sterile world into a fecund one. It is here in the marshes with the birds that I seal my relationship to Great Salt Lake.

I could never have anticipated its rise.

My mother was aware of a rise on the left side of her abdomen. I was deep in dream. This particular episode found me hiding beneath my grandmother's bed as eight black helicopters flew toward the house. I knew we were in danger.

The phone rang and everything changed.

"Good morning," I answered.

"Good morning, dear," my mother replied.

This is how my days always began. Mother and I check-ing in—a long extension cord on the telephone lets me talk and eat breakfast at the same time.

"You're back. So how was the river trip?" I asked, pouring myself a glass of orange juice.

"It was wonderful," she answered. "I loved the river and I loved the people. The Grand Canyon is a . . ."

There was a break in her voice. I set my glass on the counter.

She paused. "I didn't want to do this, Terry."

I think I knew what she was going to say before she said it. The same way, twelve years before, I knew something was wrong when I walked into our house after school and Mother was gone. In 1971, it had been breast cancer.

With my back against the kitchen wall, I slowly sank to the floor and stared at the yellow flowered wallpaper I had always intended to change.

"What I was going to say is that the Grand Canyon is a perfect place to heal—I've found a tumor, a fairly large mass in my lower abdomen. I was wondering if you could go with me to the hospital. John has to work. I'm scheduled for an ultrasound this afternoon."

I closed my eyes. "Of course."

Another pause.

"How long have you known about this?"

"I discovered it about a month ago."

I found myself getting angry until she answered the next obvious question.

"I needed time to live with it, to think about it—and more than anything else, I wanted to float down the Colorado River. This was the trip John and I had been dreaming about for years. I knew the days in the canyon would give me peace. And Terry, they did."

I sat on the white linoleum floor in my nightgown with my knees pulled in toward my chest, my head bowed.

"Maybe it's nothing, Mother. Maybe it's only a cyst. It could be benign, you know."

She did not answer.

"How do you feel?" I asked.

"I feel fine," she said. "But I would like to go shopping for a robe before my appointment at one."

We agreed to meet at eleven.

"I'm glad you're home." I said.

"So am I."

She hung up. The dial tone returned. I listened to the line until it became clear I had heard what I heard.

It's strange to feel change coming. It's easy to ignore. An underlying restlessness seems to accompany it like birds flocking before a storm. We go about our business with the usual alacrity, while in the pit of our stomach there is a sense of something tenuous.

These moments of peripheral perceptions are short, sharp flashes of insight we tend to discount like seeing the movement of an animal from the corner of our eye. We turn and there is nothing there. They are the strong and subtle impressions we allow to slip away.

I had been feeling fey for months.

Mother and I drove downtown, parked the car, and walked into Nordstrom's. I recalled the last department store we were in when the only agenda was which lipstick to choose.

We rode the escalator up two floors to sleepwear. Mother appeared to have nothing else on her mind but a beautiful piece of lingerie.

"What do you think about this one?" she asked as she held a navy blue satin robe up to her in the mirror.

"It's stunning," I answered. "I love the tiny white stars—"

"So do I. It's quite dramatic." She turned to the clerk. "I'll take this, please," and handed her the robe.

"Would you like this gift wrapped?" asked the saleswoman.

I started to say no. Mother said yes. "Thank you, that would be very nice."

My mother's flair for drama always caught me off guard. Her love of spontaneity made the most mundane enterprise an occasion. She entered a room, mystery followed her. She left and her presence lingered.

I thought of the last time we were in New York together. We slept late, rising midmorning to partake of steaming hot blueberry muffins downtown in a sidewalk café. It was my mother's sacrament. We shopped in the finest stores and twirled in front of mirrors. We lived in the museums. Having overspent our allotment of time at the Met in the Caravaggio exhibit, we opted for a quick make-over at Bloomingdale's to revive us for the theatre. The brass and glass of the department store's first floor was blinding until we finally bumped into the Lancôme counter.

"It's wonderful to be in a place where no one knows you," Mother said as she sat in the chair reserved for customers. "I would never do this at home."

The salesclerk acquainted her with options. She looked at my mother's hazel eyes, the structure of her face, her dark hair cut short.

"Great bones," the makeup artist said. "For you, less is more."

I watched the woman sweep blush across my mother's cheekbones. A hint of brown eyeshadow deepened her eyes as framboise was painted across her lips.

"How do I look?" she said.

"Dazzling," I answered.

Mother gave me her chair. The Lancôme woman looked at my face and shook her head.

"Do you spend a lot of time in the wind?"

The hospital doors seemed heavy as I pushed them open against the air trapped inside the vestibule. Once inside, it reeked of disease whitewashed with antiseptics. A trip to the hospital is always a descent into the macabre. I have never trusted a place with shiny floors.

We found our way to the lab through the maze of hallways by following the color-coded tape on the floors. Mother was given instructions to change into the hospital's blue and white seersucker robe. They say the gowns are for convenience, so they can do what they have to do fast. But their robes seem more like socialistic wraps that let you know that you belong to the fraternity of the ill waiting patiently in rooms all across America.

"Diane Tempest."

She looked too beautiful to be sick. Wearing their white foam slippers, she disappeared down the hall into a room with closed doors.

I waited.

My eyes studied each person in the room. Why were they there and what were they facing? They all seemed to share an unnatural color. I checked my hands against theirs. I tried to pick up snippets of conversation that pieced together their stories. But voices were soft and words were few.

I could not read the expression on Mother's face when she came out of X-ray. She changed into her clothes and we walked out of the hospital to the car.

"It doesn't look good," she said. "It's about the size of a

grapefruit, filled with fluid. They are calling in the results to the doctor. We need to go to his office to find out what to do next."

There was little emotion in her face. This was a time for details. Pragmatism replaced sentiment.

At Krehl Smith's office, the future was drawn on an 8½ by 11 inch pad of yellow paper. The doctor (her obstetrician who had delivered two of her four babies) proceeded to draw the tumor in relationship to her ovaries. He stumbled over his own words, not having the adequate vocabulary to tell a patient who was also a friend that she most likely had ovarian cancer.

We got the picture. There was an awkward silence.

"So what are my options?" Mother asked.

"A hysterectomy as soon as you are ready. If it is ovarian cancer then we'll follow it up with chemotherapy and go from there . . ."

"I'll make that decision," she said.

The tears I had wanted to remain hidden splashed down on the notes I was taking, blurring the ink.

Arrangements were made for surgery on Monday morning. Mother wanted to prepare the family over the weekend. Dr. Smith suggested that two oncologists be called in on the case; Gary Smith and Gary Johnson. Mother agreed, requesting that she be able to meet with them before the operation for questions.

There was another awkward silence. Details done. Mother stood up from the straight back chair.

"Thank you, Krehl."

Their eyes met. She turned to walk out the door, when Krehl Smith put his arm through hers. "I'm so sorry, Diane. I know what you went through before. I wish I had more encouraging news."

"So do I," she said. "So do I."

Mother and I got into the car. It started to rain. In a peculiar sort of way, the weather gave us permission to cry.

Driving home, Mother stared out her window. "You know, I hear the words on the outside, that I might have ovarian cancer, but they don't register on the inside. I keep saying to myself, this isn't happening to me, but then why shouldn't it? I am facing my own mortality—again—something I thought I had already done twelve years ago. Do you know how strange it is to know your days are limited? To have no future?"

Home. The family gathered in the living room. Mother had her legs on Dad's lap. Dad had his left arm around her, his right hand rubbing her knees and thighs. My brothers, Steve, Dan, and Hank were seated across the room. I sat on the hearth. A fire was burning, so were candles. Twelve years ago, we had been too young to see beyond our own pain; children of four, eight, twelve, and fifteen. Dad was thirty-seven, in shock from the thought of losing his wife. We did not do well. She did. Things were different now. We would do it together. We made promises that we would be here for her this time, that she would not have to carry us.

The conversation shifted to mountain climbing, the men's desire to climb the Grand Teton in the summer, then on to tales of scaling Mount Everest without oxygen—it could be done.

Mother said she would like to work in the garden if the weather cleared. We said we would all help.

"That's funny," she said. "No one has ever offered to help me before."

She then asked that we respect her decisions, that this was

her body and her life, not ours, and that if the tumor was malignant, she would choose not to have chemotherapy.

We said nothing.

She went on to explain why she had waited a month before going to the doctor.

"In the long run I didn't think one month would matter. In the short run, it mattered a great deal. The heat of the sandstone penetrated my skin as I lay on the red rocks. Desert light bathed my soul. And traveling through the inner gorge of Vishnu schist, the oldest exposed rock in the West, gave me a perspective that will carry me through whatever I must face. Those days on the river were a meditation, a renewal. I found my strength in its solitude. It is with me now."

She looked at Dad, "Lava Falls, John. We've got some white water ahead."

I know the solitude my mother speaks of. It is what sustains me and protects me from my mind. It renders me fully present. I am desert. I am mountains. I am Great Salt Lake. There are other languages being spoken by wind, water, and wings. There are other lives to consider: avocets, stilts, and stones. Peace is the perspective found in patterns. When I see ring-billed gulls picking on the flesh of decaying carp, I am less afraid of death. We are no more and no less than the life that surrounds us. My fears surface in my isolation. My serenity surfaces in my solitude.

It is raining. And it seems as though it has always been raining. Every day another quilted sky rolls in and covers us with water. Rain. Rain. More rain. The Great Basin is being filled.

It isn't just the clouds' doing. The depth of snowpack in the Wasatch Mountains is the highest on record. It begins to melt, and streams you could jump over become raging rivers with no place to go. Local canyons are splitting at their seams as saturated hillsides slide.

Great Salt Lake is rising.

Brooke and I opt for marriage maintenance and drive out to Black's Rock on the edge of the lake to watch birds. They'll be there in spite of the weather. And they are.

Avocets and black-necked stilts are knee-deep in water alongside Interstate 80. Flocks of California gulls stand on a disappearing beach. We pull over, get out of the car and begin walking up and over lakeside boulders. I inhale the salty air. It is like ocean, even the lake is steel-blue with whitecaps.

Brooke walks ahead while I sit down with my binoculars and watch grebes. Eared grebes. Their red eyes flash intensely on the water, and I am amazed by such buoyancy in small bodies. Scanning the horizon, all I can see is water. "Lake Bonneville," I think to myself.

It is easy to imagine this lake, born twenty-eight thousand years ago, in the Pleistocene Epoch, just one in the succession of bodies of water to inhabit the Bonneville Basin over the last fifteen million years. It inundated nearly twenty thousand square miles of western Utah, spilling into southern Utah and eastern Nevada—a liquid hand pressing against the landscape that measured 285 miles long and 140 miles wide, with an estimated depth of 1000'.

Across from where I sit, Stansbury Island looms. Distinct bench levels tell a story of old shorelines, a record of where Lake Bonneville paused in its wild fluctuations over the course of fifteen thousand years. Its rise was stalled about twenty-three thousand years ago when the lake's elevation was about 4500' above sea level; over the next three thousand years, it rose very little. The relentless erosion of wave against rock during this stable period cut a broad terrace known to geologists as the Stansbury Shoreline.

The lake began to swell again until it reached the 5090' level sixteen thousand years ago. And then for a millennium and a half, the lake carved the Bonneville Shoreline, the highest of the three main terraces. Great tongues of ice occupied canyons in the Wasatch Mountains to the east, while herds of musk oxen, mammoths, and saber-tooth cats frequented the forested shores of Lake Bonneville. Schools of Bonneville cutthroat trout flashed through these waters (remnants of which still cling to existence in the refuge of small ponds in isolated desert mountains of the Great Basin). Fossil records suggest birds similar to red-tail hawk, sage grouse, mallard, and teal lived here. And packs of dire wolves called up the moon.

About 14,500 years ago, Lake Bonneville spilled over the rim of the Great Basin near Red Rock Pass in southeastern Idaho. Suddenly, the waters broke the Basin breaching the sediments down to bedrock, releasing a flood so spectacular it is estimated the maximum discharge of water was thirty-three million cubic feet per second. This event, known today as the Bonneville Flood, dropped the lake about 350', to 4740'. When the outlet channel was eroded to resistant rock, the lake stabilized once again and the Provo Shoreline was formed.

As the climate warmed drawing moisture from the inland sea, the lake began to shrink, until, eleven thousand years ago, it had fallen to present-day levels of about 4200'. This trend toward warmer and drier conditions signified the end of the Ice Age.

A millennium later, the lake rose slightly to an elevation

of about 4250′, forming the Gilbert Shoreline, but soon receded. This marked the end of Lake Bonneville and the birth of its successor, Great Salt Lake.

As children, it was easy to accommodate the idea of Lake Bonneville. The Provo Shoreline looks like a huge bathtub ring around the Salt Lake Valley. It is a bench I know well, because we lived on it. It is the ledge that supported my neighborhood above Salt Lake City. Daily hikes in the foothills of the Wasatch yielded vast harvests of shells.

"Lake Bonneville . . ." we would say as we pocketed them. Never mind that they were the dried shells of land snails. We would sit on the benches of this ancient lake, stringing white shells into necklaces. We would look west to Great Salt Lake and imagine.

That was in 1963. I was eight years old. Great Salt Lake was a puddle, having retreated to a record low surface elevation of 4191.35′. Local papers ran headlines that read, GREAT SALT LAKE DISAPPEARING? and INLAND SEA SHRINKS.

My mother decided Great Salt Lake was something we should see before it vanished. And so, my brothers and I, with friends from the neighborhood, boarded our red Ford station wagon and headed west.

It was a long ride past the airport, industrial complexes, and municipal dumps. It was also hot. The backs of our thighs stuck to the Naugahyde seats. Our towels were wrapped around us. We were ready to swim.

Mother pulled into the Silver Sands Beach. The smell should have been our first clue, noxious hydrogen sulphide gas rising from the brine.

"Phew!" we all complained as we walked toward the beach, brine flies following us. "Smells like rotten eggs."

"You'll get used to it," Mother said. "Now go play. See if you can float."

We were dubious at best. Our second clue should have

been the fact that Mother did not bring her bathing suit, but rather chose to sit on the sand in her sunsuit with a thick novel in hand.

The ritual was always the same. Run into the lake, scream, and run back out. The salt seeped into the sores of our scraped knees and lingered. And if the stinging sensation didn't bring you to tears, the brine flies did.

We huddled around Mother, the old Saltair Pavilion was visible behind her, vibrating behind a screen of heatwaves. We begged her to take us home, pleading for dry towels. Total time at the lake: five minutes. She was unsympathetic.

"We're here for the afternoon, kids," she said, and then brought down her sunglasses a bit so we could see her eyes. "I didn't see anyone floating."

She had given us a dare. One by one, we slowly entered Great Salt Lake. Gradually, we would lean backward into the hands of the cool water and find ourselves being held by the very lake that minutes before had betrayed us. For hours we floated on our backs, imprinting on Great Basin skies. It was in these moments of childhood that Great Salt Lake flooded my psyche.

Driving home, Mother asked each of us what we thought of the lake. None of us said much. We were too preoccupied with our discomfort: sunburned and salty, we looked like red gumdrops. Our hair felt like steel wool, and we smelled. With the lake so low and salinity around 26 percent, one pound of salt to every four pounds of water (half a gallon), another hour of floating in Great Salt Lake and we might have risked being pickled and cured.

Brooke brought me back a handful of feathers and sat behind me. I leaned back into his arms. Three more days until Mother's surgery.

The family spontaneously gathered at Mother's and Dad's; children, spouses, grandparents, and cousins. We sat on the lawn, some talked, others played gin rummy, while Mother planted marigolds in her garden.

Mother and I talked.

"I don't want you to be disappointed, Terry."

"I won't be," I said softly. My hands patted the earth around each flower she planted.

"It's funny how the tears finally leave you," she said, turning her trowel in the soil. "I think I've experienced every possible emotion this week."

"And how do you feel now?" I asked.

She looked out at the lake, wiped her forehead with the back of her gardening glove, and removed more marigolds from the flat.

"I'll be glad to have the operation behind me. I'm ready to get on with my life."

Dad mowed the lawn between clumps of relatives. It felt good to be outside, to feel the heat, and to hear the sounds of neighborhoods on Saturdays in the spring.

The sun set behind Antelope Island. Great Salt Lake was a mirror on the valley floor. One had the sense of water being in this country now, as the quality of light was different lending a high gloss to the foothills.

At dusk, we moved inside to the living room and created a family circle. Mother sat on a chair in the center. As the eldest son, Steve annointed Mother with consecrated olive oil to seal the blessing. The men who held the Melchizedek Priesthood, the highest order of authority bestowed upon Mormon males, gathered around her, placing their hands on the crown of her head. My father prayed in a low, humble voice, asking that she might be the receptacle of her family's love, that she might know of her influence in our lives and be blessed with strength and courage and peace of mind.

Kneeling next to my grandmother, Mimi, I felt her strength and the generational history of belief Mormon ritual holds. We can heal ourselves, I thought, and we can heal each other.

"These things we pray for in the name of Jesus Christ, amen."

Mother opened her eyes. "Thank you . . ."

My sister-in-law, Ann, and I slipped into the kitchen to prepare dinner.

Some things don't change. After everyone had eaten, attention shifted to the weather report on the ten o'clock news, a Western ritual, especially when your livelihood depends on it as ours does. A family construction business, now in its fourth generation, has taught me to look up before I look down. You can't lay pipe when the ground is frozen, neither can you have crews digging trenches in mud.

The weatherman not only promised good weather, but announced that most of the planet would be clear tomorrow according to the satellite projection—a powerful omen in itself.

After everyone left, I asked Mother if I could feel the tumor. She lay down on the carpet in the family room and placed my hand on her abdomen. With her help, I found the strange rise on the left side and palpated my fingers around its perimeter.

With my hands on my mother's belly, I prayed.

We wait. Our family is pacing the hall. Other families are pacing other halls. Each tragedy has its own territory. A Tongan family in the room next to Mother's sings mourning songs for the dying. Their melancholy sweeps over us like the shadow of a raven. What songs would we sing, I wonder. Two doors down, a nurse calls for assistance in turning a patient over on a bed of ice. Minutes later, I hear the groaning of the chilled woman.

It has been almost four hours. For most of the time, I have been sitting with my mother's parents. My grandmother, Lettie, is in a wheelchair. She suffers from Parkinson's disease. Her delicate hands tremble as she strokes my hair. I am leaning against the side of her knee. She and my grandfather, Sanky, are heartsick. Mother is their only daughter; one of their two sons is dead. Mother has always cared for her parents. Now that she needs their help, Lettie feels the pain of a mother unable to physically attend to her daughter.

The three doctors appear: Smith, Smith, and Johnson, green-robed and capped. Dad meets them halfway, cowboy boots toe-to-toe with surgical papered shoes. I try to read lips as he receives the bad news followed by the good news.

"Yes, it was malignant. No we didn't get it all, but with the chemotherapy we have to offer, there is reason to be hopeful." The doctors say they will meet with us in a couple of days when they get the pathology report back, then they will go over specific details and options with Mother and the family.

Dad—tall, rugged, and direct—asks one question. "What's the bottom line—how much time do we have?"

The doctors meet his narrow blue eyes. Gary Smith shakes his head. "We can't tell you that. No one can."

The curse and charisma of cancer: the knowledge that from this point forward, all you have is the day at hand.

Dad turned around defeated, frustrated. "I'd like to get some answers." His impatience became his stride as he walked back down the hall.

Bad news is miraculously accommodated. With one hope dashed—the tumor was malignant (an easier word to stomach than cancer)—another hope is adopted: the chemotherapy will cure. Now all we had to do was convince Mother. We made a pact among ourselves that we would not discuss anything with her until the next morning. We wanted her to rest.

Two orderlies wheel Mother back into her room. The tubes, bags, blood, and lines dangling from four directions did not foster the hope we were trying to sustain. Our faith faltered in the presence of her face—white, wan, and weakened. Dad whispered that she looked like a skinned deer.

Mother opened her eyes and faintly chuckled, "That bad, uh?"

No one else laughed. We just looked at one another. We were awkward and ill-prepared.

Dad took Mother's hand and spoke to her reassuringly. He tried stroking her arm but quickly became frustrated and frightened by all the tubing connected to her veins. He sat with her as long as he could maintain his composure and then retreated to the hall where his parents, Mimi and Jack, were standing by.

Steve, Dan, and Hank took over, each one nursing her in his own way.

"Don't worry about fixing dinner for Dad tonight, Mom, we'll take care of him," said Steve.

Dan walked out of the room and came back with a cup of ice chips. "Would you like to suck on these, Mother? Your mouth looks dry."

Hank, sixteen, stood in the corner and watched. Mother looked at him and extended her hand. He walked toward her and took it.

"Love you, Mom."

"I love you, too, dear," she whispered.

My brothers left the room. I stood at the foot of her bed, "How are you feeling, Mother?"

It was a hollow question, I knew, but words don't count when words don't matter. I moved to her side and stroked her forehead. Her eyes pierced mine.

"Did they get it all?"

I blinked and looked away.

"Did they, Terry? Tell me." She grabbed my hand.

I shook my head. "No, Mother."

She closed her eyes and I watched the muscles in her jaw tighten.

"How bad is it?"

Dad walked in and saw the tears streaming down my cheeks. "What happened?"

I shook my head again, left the room and walked down the hall. He followed me and took hold of my shoulder.

"You didn't tell her, did you?"

I turned around, still crying, and faced him. "Yes."

"Why? Why, when we agreed not to say anything until tomorrow? It wasn't your place." His anger flared like the corona of an eclipsed sun.

"I told her because she asked me, and I could not lie."

The pathologist's report defined Mother's tumor as Stage III epithelial ovarian cancer. It had metastasized to the abdominal cavity. Nevertheless, Dr. Gary Smith believes Mother has a very good chance against this type of cancer, given the treatment available. He is recommending one year of chemotherapy using the agents Cytoxan and cisplatin.

Before surgery, Mother said no chemotherapy.

Today, I walked into her room, the blinds were closed. "Terry," she said through the darkness. "Will you help me? I told myself I would not let them poison me. But now I am afraid not to. I want to live."

I sat down by her bed.

"Perhaps you can help me visualize a river—I can imagine the chemotherapy to be a river running through me, flushing the cancer cells out. Which river, Terry?"

"How about the Colorado?" I said.

It was the first time in weeks I had seen my mother smile.

June 1, 1983. Mayor Ted Wilson has ordered the channeling of three mountain streams, Red Butte, Emigration, and Parley's, into a holding pond at Liberty Park near the center of town. From Liberty Park, the water will be funneled into the Jordan River, which will eventually pour into Great Salt Lake.

Normally, these three Wasatch Front rivers converge underground in an eighty-inch pipe, but when the pipe gets too full, it blows all the manhole covers sky high, causing massive flooding on the streets. It's called "Project Earthworks."

Yesterday's temperature was sixty-two degrees Fahrenheit. Today it is ninety-two. All hell is about to break loose in the mountains. A quick thaw is a quick flood.

Ten days have passed and, between all of us, we have kept vigil. Mother's strength is returning and with typical wit, she hinted that a bit of privacy might be nice. I took her cue and drove out to the Bird Refuge.

It looked like any other spring. Western kingbirds lined the fences, their yellow bellies flashing bright above the barbed wire. Avocets and stilts were still occupying the same shallow ponds they had always inhabited, and the white-faced glossy ibises six miles from the Refuge were meticulously separating the grasses with their decurved bills.

Closer in, the alkaline flats, usually dry, stark, and vacant, were wet. A quarter mile out, they were flooded.

The Bear River Migratory Bird Refuge, at an elevation of 4206′, was two feet from being inundated. I walked out as far as I could. It had been a long time since I had heard the liquid songs of red-wing blackbirds.

"Konk-la-ree! Konk-la-ree! Konk-la-ree!"

The marsh was flooding. The tips of cattails looked like snorkels jutting a few inches above water. Coots' nests floated. They would fare well. With my binoculars, I could see snowy egrets fishing the small cascades that were breaking over the road's asphalt shoulders.

I could not separate the Bird Refuge from my family. Devastation respects no boundaries. The landscape of my childhood and the landscape of my family, the two things I had always regarded as bedrock, were now subject to change. Quicksand.

Looking out over the water, now an ocean, I felt foolish for standing in the middle of what little road was left. Better to have brought a canoe. But I rolled up my pantlegs over the tops of my rubber boots and continued to walk. I knew my ground.

Up ahead, two dozen white pelicans were creating a spiral staircase as they flew. It looked like a feathered DNA molecule. Their wings reflected the sun. The light shifted, and they disappeared. It shifted again and I found form. Escher's inspiration. The pelicans rose higher and higher on black-tipped wings until they straightened themselves into an arrow pointing west to Gunnison Island.

To my left, long-billed dowitchers, stout and mottled

birds, pattered and probed, pattered and probed, perforating the mud in masses. In an instant, they flew, sweeping the sky as one great bird. Flock consciousness.

I turned away from the water and walked east toward the mountains. Foxtails by the roadside gathered light and held it. Dry stalks of rumex, russet from last year's fall, drew hunger pangs—the innocence of those days.

Before leaving, I noticed sago pondweed screening shallow water near the edge of the road. Tiny green circles of chlorophyll were converting sunlight to sugar. I knelt down and scooped up a handful. Microscopic animals and a myriad of larvae drained from my hands. Within seconds, the marsh in microcosm slipped through my fingers.

I was not prepared for the loneliness that followed.

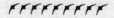

SNOWY EGRETS

lake level: 4204.05'

I caught myself staring out the window again. Last time I looked at the clock it was 11:20 A.M. Now it is 12:30.

From my third floor office at the Utah Museum of Natural History, I look out over roofs and watch a pair of kestrels flying in and out of the cottonwoods. They have a nest nearby. Beyond them loom the Wasatch. Their peaks still hold the snow in early summer.

I was with Mother yesterday during her first chemotherapy treatment. Her fear and resistance did not help. Resignation, I suppose, would be worse. I held her forehead as she writhed, wretched, and heaved. She would cry and I would cry with her. I just kept saying, "Let it go, Mother, we'll get through this." At one point, after the nurses left, I got into bed with her and held her close to absorb her trembling body. She was so cold, even blankets wouldn't help. Dr.

Smith said the first treatment is the most severe, especially since she is still recovering from the surgery.

My desk is heaped high with papers, pink notes, and mail; bureaucratic accumulation from my "vacation time."

The phone rings—I don't answer.

My eyes focus on a plate full of shells I brought home from Mexico. It has sat on my windowsill during the three years I have worked here. I pull the crab claw out from under the pink murex. It repulses me. This is cancer, my mother's process, not mine.

The disengaged limb holds me, haunts me. I can't let it go. There is something in my resistance that warrants attention.

Cancer. The word has infinite power. It kills us with its name first, because we have allowed it to become synonymous with death.

The Oxford English Dictionary defines cancer as "anything that frets, corrodes, corrupts, or consumes slowly and secretly."

A person who is told she has cancer faces a hideous recognition that something monstrous is happening within her own body.

Cancer becomes a disease of shame, one that encourages secrets and lies, to protect as well as to conceal.

And then suddenly, within the rooms of secrecy, patient, doctor, and family find themselves engaged in war. Once again, medical language is loaded, this time with military metaphors: the fight, the battle, enemy infiltration, and defense strategies. I wonder if this kind of aggression waged against our own bodies is counterproductive to healing? Can we be at war with ourselves and still find peace?

How can we rethink cancer?

It begins slowly and is largely hidden. One cell divides

into two; two cells divide into four; four cells divide into sixteen . . . normal cells are consumed by abnormal ones. Over time, they congeal, consolidate, make themselves known. Call it a mass, call it a tumor. It surfaces and demands our attention. We can surgically remove it. We can shrink it with radiation. We can poison it with drugs. Whatever we choose, though, we view the tumor as foreign, something outside ourselves. It is however, our own creation. The creation we fear.

The cancer process is not unlike the creative process. Ideas emerge slowly, quietly, invisibly at first. They are most often abnormal thoughts, thoughts that disrupt the quotidian, the accustomed. They divide and multiply, become invasive. With time, they congeal, consolidate, and make themselves conscious. An idea surfaces and demands total attention. I take it from my body and give it away.

I pick up the crab claw and put it in my pocket. I can hardly wait to tell Mother.

The phone rings again—this time I answer.

"Museum education, may I help you?"

It is someone calling about the upcoming film series entitled "The Gentle Earth," a confirmation that Toby McLeod's film, "Four Corners: A National Sacrifice Area," is available for a Salt Lake City premiere.

Good news. But I need to convince our director that it is in the museum's best interest to sponsor a film about uranium tailings in Navajoland. Nothing inspires me more than a little controversy. We are in the business of waking people up to their surroundings. A museum is a good place to be quietly subversive on behalf of the land.

I close my door and begin to plot my strategy.

Downtown; the North Temple storm pipe that han-
dles City Creek had been doing fine all week in spite of an
increase in water flow from an average 50 cubic feet per
second to 375 cubic feet per second. (The previous record
was 90 cubic feet per second.) But the rocks, silt, and debris
had caused a dense mass like concrete to form. The water
had had no place to go and, consequently, it was backing
up onto city streets. Mountain Bell Communications Systems and the LDS Church Office Building were in immediate danger of flooding.

The mayor, Ted Wilson, telephoned President Gordon B.
Hinckley, an apostle of the Mormon Church. His request:
"Empty the ward houses."

"But it's the sabbath—" Hinckley replied.

"We need your help. City Creek has literally become
unglued, and a two foot wall of water is charging through
Memory Grove. The Church Office Building could be next.
Your genealogical records . . ." Within ten minutes, Mormon chapels across the Salt Lake Valley were vacated.

"Go home and change your clothes—we've got a flood
on our hands . . ." was the message given over the pulpit.

Mayor Wilson received a call back from Hinckley.

"The ox is in the mire."

By 2:00 P.M., thousands of volunteers with their shirt-
sleeves rolled up, Mormons and non-Mormons alike, lined
State Street, which runs north and south for miles down the
heart of the city. Within hours, State Street was transformed
into a river.

Ted Wilson, on the news last night called it "a victimless
war." Mother and I watched it from her hospital room,
knowing the men in our family were part of the community
throng building the three-foot walls of sandbags.

Dad, Steve, Dan, and Hank wandered in around ten o'clock in muddy Levi's and great spirits. Brooke followed shortly after.

"You should see it on the streets, Diane!" Dad said. "It's incredible. Sandbags were delivered. The city engineers had envisioned the plan, but there was no midlevel management to execute it."

"So, let me guess," I chided Dad, "you became General Patton."

"Not exactly," he said smiling, "but sort of. We made a line from the truck to the street, sandbags being passed left to right, left to right, for what seemed like hours. Then the volunteers on the street judged the grade and built the banks accordingly. Everyone brought their own ideas how it could best be done. There was total cooperation."

Dad sat down on the edge of Mother's hospital bed. "When the water was finally released from City Creek and began flowing down State Street, you should have heard the cheers. Cries from the crowd followed the water block after block like a wave.

"All I know," said Hank, "is that it was a great way to get out of church."

The sandbag banks held City Creek for almost three miles. In some places, the water was three feet deep. Where cars once drove, fish swam. Where pedestrians once crossed, bridges now spanned. A car bridge between the city blocks of 500 and 600 South was erected for the price of seventy thousand dollars—no small risk financially, for a mayor who saw his town being truncated, cut in half by flooding and not having a clue how long it might last. But his hunch paid off. The city kept moving in spite of the floods. And the State Street River kept flowing.

The flooding of Salt Lake City lifted everyone's spirits. People went fishing. Signs saying YOU CATCH 'EM—WE'LL

COOK 'EM were posted in front of State Street restaurants. A few trout were caught and fried.

A bride and groom exchanged vows on the bridge. They later walked arm in arm into the Alta Club for their wedding breakfast. A crowd followed them throwing rice.

My favorite innovations were made by the kayakers who complained about having to portage around the city-block bridges and made local officials promise to build rialtos next time with appropriate clearance. Class-three rapids were reported between South Temple and 100 South.

July 1, 1983. Great Salt Lake has risen 5.1' since September 18, 1982, the greatest seasonal rise ever recorded. And it's still rising. Hal Cannon, a folklorist, and I drive out to the Bird Refuge to see how the marsh is faring. We decided to swap expertise: he would fill me in on noteworthy collectibles at the Deseret Industries, a Mormon thrift shop, if I would take him to Bear River to watch birds.

Inside the Deseret Industries in Brigham City, Hal looks for glass grapes, any color. They were made by every Mormon woman in Relief Society, the women's auxiliary organization, during the 1960s (my own mother included). Boxes of glass balls were set on top of banquet tables in the Cultural Hall. You could pick your color and size. Turquoise, amber, red, and purple seemed to be the most popular. And then you could choose from dainty glass grapes to balls the size of silver dollars. Each woman was provided with a stick, which served as the bunch stalk. These were painted brown, then shellacked. Green leaves made out of silk were added next with copper wires curled into tendrils. The last step was to glue the glass balls together until you had your bunch of grapes. This seemed to be where the women ran into problems—they didn't know when to stop. Some of the glass ball masterpieces flowed halfway down the tables, looking like mutant clusters of salmon eggs. The women ended up carrying them to their cars in both hands. Coffee tables at home were in danger of collapsing under their weight. Every home had one, whether the women liked them or not. It was a symbol of craft adeptness, an important tenet of Mormonism.

Mother wasn't great with crafts. Her grapes, an amber cluster with glass balls the size of quarters, were modest.

"I was just glad to get it done so I could go home," I remember her saying. Nevertheless, they stayed on the bookshelf in the kitchen for years, until dust finally obscured their luster and a new fad like gingham geese replaced them.

No grapes are to be found on this trip to the Deseret Industries. Instead, Hal finds an old tweed coat that fits his husky frame like a glove. I splurge and buy a pink cashmere sweater with pearled and sequined flowers down the front for five dollars.

We drive through the flooding Bird Refuge in Hal's turquoise Comet convertible. It is the perfect birdwatching vehicle. Dozens of avocets and stilts fly over us, flocks of ibises fly alongside. Gulls are everywhere. I love seeing their bellies. (Hal reminds me we need umbrellas.) We are in an avian parade traveling west. I threaten to crawl into the back seat, perch on top of the trunk, and make figure eight waves to all the marsh like a float queen.

Luckily, two snowy egrets fly over us and distract me. My dignity is preserved.

We park the car and walk to the edge of cattails. Hunkering down, we separate the stalks with our fingers and find the egrets. I nudge Hal. One egret spears a small frog. A blink and we would have missed it. We watch them walk along the periphery of the pond in their "golden slippers." Snowy egrets have yellow feet.

We have lost track of time in a birdwatchers' trance. Egret plumes like French lace billow in the breeze and underscore their amorous play. One egret rises, the other follows. Their steps are light and buoyant. Hal leans toward me and softly hums an Irish folktune. The two egrets stagger their leaps—one lifts, one lands, one lifts, one lands—and the dance continues.

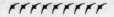

BARN SWALLOWS

lake level: 4204.75'

What is it about the relationship of a mother that can heal or hurt us? Her womb is the first landscape we inhabit. It is here we learn to respond—to move, to listen, to be nourished and grow. In her body we grow to be human as our tails disappear and our gills turn to lungs. Our maternal environment is perfectly safe—dark, warm, and wet. It is a residency inside the Feminine.

When we outgrow our mother's body, our cramps become her own. We move. She labors. Our body turns upside down in hers as we journey through the birth canal. She pushes in pain. We emerge, a head. She pushes one more time, and we slide out like a fish. Slapped on the back by the doctor, we breathe. The umbilical cord is cut—not at our request. Separation is immediate. A mother reclaims her body, for her own life. Not ours. Minutes old, our first death is our own birth.

Mother and I are in Wyoming. The quaking aspens
are ablaze like the bright light of a burning match. We walk
along the Gros Ventre River with the Tetons behind us. She
gave me my birth story: what she experienced during her
pregnancy, what the birthing was like, and how she felt
when she held me for the first time.

"I don't ever remember being so happy, Terry. Having
a child completed something for me. I can't explain it.
It's something you feel as a woman connected to other
women."

She paused.

I asked her if she thought my life was selfish without
children.

"Yes," she said. "But I'm not saying that's bad. By being
selfish a woman ultimately has more to give in the long run,
because she has a self to give away."

"Do you think I should have a child?" I asked.

"I can't answer that for you," she said. "All I can tell you
is that it was the right choice for me."

Across the river, Mother and I watch two elk. Bulls in
the midst of their harems. She says they are eating. I say their
antlers are locked and they are sparring.

"You have the most vivid imagination," she says. "Let me
see your binoculars." She pulls them up to her eyes. "Okay,
I'll give you this one."

Walking back to our family's place, we are seized by the
alpenglow, a cradle of pink light. The willows are rust and
maroon, the mountains purple. Trumpeter swans float above
their reflections on the river. A pair of bald eagles fly across
the face of the Tetons. Their heads seemed brighter than the
promise of snow.

The next day, we awake at dawn and travel once again
down to the river bottoms. We watch a herd of pronghorn

antelope grazing on the moraine. A buck flares his fanny at us.

"Am I imagining this one?" I turn to Mother and hand her the binoculars.

"Do you blame him?" Mother replies. "We are beautiful women."

This afternoon, I have found quiet hours alone picking tomatoes. As my fingers find ripe tomatoes, red and firm, through the labyrinth of leaves, I am absorbed into the present. My garden asks nothing more of me than I am able to give. I pull tomatoes, gently placing them in the copper colander. Pulling tomatoes. Pulling tomatoes. Some come easily.

Tonight I watched the sun sink behind the lake. The clouds looked like rainbow trout swimming in a lapis sky. I can honor its beauty or resent the smog in this valley which makes it possible. Either way, I am deceiving myself.

Mother has completed her sixth month of chemotherapy. In some ways, it is easy to become complacent, to take life for granted all over again. I welcome this luxury. I have the feeling Mother is living in the heart of each day. I am not.

Buddha says there are two kinds of suffering: the kind that leads to more suffering and the kind that brings an end to suffering.

I recall a barn swallow who had somehow wrapped his tiny leg around the top rung of a barbed-wire fence. I was walking the dikes at Bear River. When I saw the bird, my first instinct was to stop and help. But then, I thought, no, there is nothing I can do, the swallow is going to die. But I could not leave the bird. I finally took it in my hands and unwrapped it from the wire. Its heart was racing against my fingers. The swallow had exhausted itself. I placed it among the blades of grass and sat a few feet away. With each breath, it threw back its head, until the breaths grew fainter and fainter. The tiny chest became still. Its eyes were half closed. The barn swallow was dead.

Suffering shows us what we are attached to—perhaps the umbilical cord between Mother and me has never been cut. Dying doesn't cause suffering. Resistance to dying does.

PEREGRINE FALCON

lake level: 4205.40'

Not far from Great Salt Lake is the municipal dump. Acres of trash heaped high. Depending on your frame of mind, it is either an olfactory fright show or a sociological gold mine. Either way, it is best to visit in winter.

For the past few years, when the Christmas Bird Count comes around, I seem to be relegated to the landfill. The local Audubon hierarchy tell me I am sent there because I know gulls. The truth lies deeper. It's an under-the-table favor. I am sent to the dump because secretly they know I like it.

As far as birding goes, there's often no place better. Our urban wastelands are becoming wildlife's last stand. The great frontier. We've moved them out of town like all other "low-income tenants."

The dump where I count birds for Christmas used to have cattails—but I can't remember them. A few have popped up below the hill again, in spite of the bulldozers, providing critical cover for coots, mallards, and a variety of other waterfowl. I've seen herons standing by and once a snowy egret, but for the most part, the habitat now is garbage, perfect for starlings and gulls.

I like to sit on the piles of unbroken Hefties, black bubbles of sanitation. It provides comfort with a view. Thousands of starlings cover refuse with their feet. Everywhere I look—feathered trash.

The starlings gorge themselves, bumping into each other like drunks. They are not discretionary. They'll eat anything, just like us. Three starlings picked a turkey carcass clean. Afterward, they crawled inside and wore it as a helmet. A carcass with six legs walking around—you have to be sharp counting birds at the dump.

I admire starlings' remarkable adaptability. Home is everywhere. I've seen them nesting under awnings on New York's Fifth Avenue, as well as inside aspen trunks in the Teton wilderness. Over 50 percent of their diet is insects. They are the most effective predators against the clover weevil in America.

Starlings are also quite beautiful if looked at with beginner's eyes. In autumn and winter, their plumage appears speckled, unkempt. But by spring, the lighter tips of their feathers have been worn away, leaving them with a black, glossy plumage, glistening with irridescences.

Inevitably, students at the museum will describe an elegant, black bird with flashes of green, pink, and purple.

"About this big," they say (holding their hands about seven inches apart vertically). "With a bright yellow bill. What is it?"

"A starling," I answer.

What follows is a dejected look flushed with embarrassment.

"Is that all?"

The name precedes the bird.

I understand it. When I'm out at the dump with starlings, I don't want to like them. They are common. They are aggressive, and they behave poorly, crowding out other birds. When a harrier happens to cross over from the marsh, they swarm him. He disappears. They want their trash to themselves.

Perhaps we project on to starlings that which we deplore in ourselves: our numbers, our aggression, our greed, and our cruelty. Like starlings, we are taking over the world.

The parallels continue. Starlings forage by day in open country competing with native species such as bluebirds for food. They drive them out. In late afternoon, they return in small groups to nest elsewhere, competing with cavity nesters such as flickers, martins, tree swallows, and chickadees. Once again, they move in on other birds' territories.

Starlings are sophisticated mimics singing songs of bobwhites, killdeer, flickers, and phoebes. Their flocks drape bare branches in spring with choruses of chatters, creeks, and coos. Like any good impostor, they confuse the boundaries. They lie.

What is the impact of such a species on the land? Quite simply, a loss of diversity.

What makes our relationship to starlings even more curious is that we loathe them, calling in exterminators because we fear disease, yet we do everything within our power to encourage them as we systematically erase the specialized habitats of specialized birds. I have yet to see a snowy egret spearing a bagel.

The man who wanted Shakespeare's birds flying in Central Park and altruistically brought starlings to America from England, is not to blame. We are—for creating more and more habitat for a bird we despise. Perhaps the only value in the multitudes of starlings we have garnished is that in some small way they allow us to comprehend what vast flocks of birds must have felt like.

The symmetry of starling flocks takes my breath away; I lose track of time and space. At the dump, all it takes is the sweep of my hand. They rise. Hundreds of starlings. They wheel and turn, twist and glide, with no apparent leader. They are the collective. A flight of frenzy. They are black stars against a blue sky. I watch them above the dump, expanding and contracting along the meridian of a winged universe.

Suddenly, the flock pulls together like a winced eye, then opens in an explosion of feathers. A peregrine falcon is expelled, but not without its prey. With folded wings he strikes a starling and plucks its body from mid-air. The flock blinks again and the starlings disperse, one by one, returning to the landfill.

The starlings at the Salt Lake City municipal dump give us numbers that look good on our Christmas Bird Count, thousands, but they become faceless when compared to one peregrine falcon. A century ago, he would have seized a teal.

I will continue to count birds at the dump, hoping for under-the-table favors, but don't mistake my motives. I am not contemplating starlings. It is the falcon I wait for—the duckhawk with a memory for birds that once blotted out the sun.

WILSON'S PHALAROPE

ℱℱℱℱℱℱℱℱ

lake level: 4206.15'

In 1975, the Utah State Legislature passed a law stating Great
Salt Lake could not exceed 4202'. Almost ten years later, at
lake level 4206.15', Great Salt Lake is above the law. What
lasso can you use to corral the West's latest outlaw?

The State of Utah is reviewing its options to control the
lake. They have come up with five alternatives:

Option One: Breaching the Causeway
The Southern Pacific Railroad Causeway, built in 1957,
divides Great Salt Lake in two, running west from Promontory Point to the Lakeside Mountains. The rock-fill structure spans almost thirteen miles. All freshwater inflow to the
lake enters the lake's south arm. Two fifteen-foot culverts
located in the middle of the causeway allow water to move
from the south arm to the north, but at a rate much lower
than that of the inflow to the south arm. Consequently, the

elevation difference between the south and north arms of Great Salt Lake is almost four feet. For this reason, the salinity in the southern arm is less, which affects the brine shrimp and algae populations.

If the causeway were breached with a larger opening, the level of the south arm could be reduced by one foot, buying enough time for the wet weather to subside and allowing Great Salt Lake to flow back to its original shape.

Estimated cost: $3,000,000.

Option Two: Store the Water
If there's a water problem in the West, build a dam. The Bear River is the largest tributary of Great Salt Lake, responsible for 60 percent of all stream inflow. Dam it. Store it. Create a reservoir. Nine different reservoir sites are under consideration, but preliminary studies reveal the maximum possible storage would yield only three hundred thousand acre-feet and have only a minimal effect on the flooding problems.

Estimated cost: $100,000,000 plus.

Option Three: Divert the Water
Since the Bear River was diverted from the Snake River by a volcanic dam some twenty million years ago, why not simply reroute it back to its original path? Never mind the politics of water rights, state boundaries, and engineering logistics.

Estimated cost: $200,000,000.

Option Four: Diking
Protective diking along the shore of Great Salt Lake, from the town of Corrine in Box Elder County to the north to Interstate 80 in Tooele County south, seems like a logical solution.

Estimated cost: $500,000,000 plus.

Selective diking as a short-term solution to protect critical public facilities such as wastewater treatment plants, interstate highways, and the airport, is already underway.

A second diking concept, a long-term solution, would build a dike on the existing causeway which connects the northern end of Antelope Island to the mainland community of Syracuse. A second dike would connect the southern tip of Antelope Island to Interstate 80.

Other interisland diking would include linking Promontory Point, Fremont Island, and Antelope Island—a dot-to-dot exercise in hydrological engineering.

This project would require a large pumping plant to remove the inflows of the Bear, Weber, and Jordan Rivers so that an acceptable water level in the impounded areas could be maintained.

Estimated cost: $250,000,000.

Option Five: West Desert Pumping Project

Originally Brigham Young's idea, it was first investigated by the Army Corps of Engineers in 1976. The plan proposed to dike off Great Salt Lake near Lakeside (on the western shore of the lake) and pump water over the dike, letting it flow naturally into the West Desert. It was determined unfeasible because it threatened the United States Air Force bombing range. We would be flooding a critical national defense facility.

A pumping project would have to be devised that would lift lake water over Hogup Mountain Ridge, to the desert west of the Newfoundland Mountains, causing only minimal effect on the bombing reservation. This would mean the water would have to be released high enough so that it could flow by gravity into an evaporation pond, and then back again to Great Salt Lake.

The West Desert Pumping Project is being looked at as an extreme measure in the event that the unprecedented wet period continues into subsequent years.

Estimated cost: $90,000,000.

It was decided after much debate on the House and Senate floors that breaching the Southern Pacific Railroad Causeway would give the most immediate relief for the least money.

House Bill 30 was passed, which provides $3.5 million dollars to construct a three-hundred-foot opening. The contract is to begin immediately.

Evidently, to do nothing is not an option.

"If someone would have told me one year ago, I would be going through eleven months of chemotherapy for ovarian cancer, I would never have believed them," Mother said. "Now that it's over—I don't know how I managed. It's funny what you can will yourself through when you have to."

We were on our way to lunch to celebrate Mother's birthday. March 7, 1932. She was fifty-two years old.

"What would you tell your children of me?" Mother asked after we had seated ourselves in the restaurant at Hotel Utah.

I unfolded my napkin and placed it on my lap. I didn't want to think about such things.

"I'll let you tell them for yourself," I answered, taking a sip of water.

She paused and placed her napkin on her lap.

"Tell them I am the bird's nest behind the waterfall. Yes, tell them that."

Great Salt Lake has swallowed the causeway that led to Antelope Island. Gone. The road has been erased. Gentle waves cross over each other from north and south. A sign half submerged reads, SPEED LIMIT 45 m.p.h. It must apply to the birds. Thirty miles to the north, the Bird Refuge is underwater.

Three men from Parks and Recreation are removing the last boat slips. I'm sitting on one of the wooden frames as the crane removes others to my left. I ask if I am bothering them.

"You can sit out here as long as you like, lady," the foreman replies. "In fact, you can walk out as far as your heart will carry you . . ."

The men go about their business. Ten white pelicans glide over us, their wing beats slow and deliberate. One of the men looks up, looks at me, and raises his eyebrows. Five avocets fly north. A cluster of cinnamon teals wing south. Coots, eared grebes, and gulls float on the lake as Wilson's phalaropes pirouette in the water.

The men look bored with their work. One of the workers looks over his shoulder and throws two wooden slats in a pile.

"Did you know the female phalarope, the small bird between the slips, wears the bright plumage in this species, not the male?"

No one comments.

"And see how she keeps twirling around?" I say, keeping my binoculars on the birds.

"Let me guess . . ." replies one of the men. "Someone wound it up and lost the key."

"It's their way of stirring up food lodged at the bottom of the lake. Their feet create a whirlwind from which they can feed. They don't take in as much salt that way either.

I've even heard that some phalaropes have been seen spinning at sixty revolutions per minute."

"Who in the hell would spend their life counting how many times a bird spins around?" one of the men asks incredulously.

"That's what I do for a living," I said.

The three men stop working and stare. This time, I laugh. "So, what do you really think about the governor wanting to build a new causeway to the island?"

"Me?" asks the employee who noticed the pelicans. "I just work here."

I tell him his eyes don't look like he just works here.

He grins. He reminds me of my brothers.

"Between you and me, they ought to just let the lake do its thing. It will anyway. It always does. They can come back and rebuild the road on another day when it decides to recede."

He pauses after he finishes breaking up some asphalt. "It changes out here every week. In January, you could drive out to the island. Now, well, now you need a boat or wings," he says, chuckling. "And where you stand today, a week from now you would be knee-deep in brine."

Another worker agrees. "Last month, this was all mud-flats. Every day we watch the lake eat another chunk of the road."

"You never know what you're going to find out here. Last February, I saw icebergs the size of pickup trucks floating on the lake. And a month from now, it'll be a buggy nightmare. This lake attracts flies like a magnet attracts iron shavings. Best to go home, it's so hot and miserable."

The foreman adds, "Boil or freeze at the Great Salt Lake, and if the weather doesn't kill you, the brine flies will . . ." He hums to a tune from the Grateful Dead.

Two curlews fly overhead. Three great blue herons,

evenly spaced, fish along shore. As I hop down from the boat slip, the lake laps around my ankles.

The foreman turns around. "No matter what they tell you on the news, the lake's still risin'."

I leave the men at the causeway and find a more remote vantage point of Antelope Island on dry ground. From where I sit now, it looks like a large buckskinned animal sleeping on its side. The rural country with monarchs on milkweeds on the eastern shore of Great Salt Lake almost allows me to believe this is a calm and predictable place.

I watch the island intently with my binoculars, scanning the shoreline, noticing where beaches end and outcroppings of stone begin. The island appears still and serene, but I know better. Buffalo live here. I have also seen deer and coyotes. Vultures clip the ridgelines in search of carrion, and the wind is always present. But in spite of the human hand, Antelope Island remains remarkably pristine. A state park claims the northern tip with a few facilities for tourists, but with the causeway submerged, it becomes wild and uninterrupted country once again.

The pulse of Great Salt Lake, surging along Antelope Island's shores, becomes the force wearing against my mother's body. And when I watch flocks of phalaropes wing their way toward quiet bays on the island, I recall watching Mother sleep, imagining the dreams that were encircling her, wondering what she knows that I must learn for myself. The light changes, Antelope Island is blue. Mother awakened and I looked away.

Antelope Island is no longer accessible to me. It is my mother's body floating in uncertainty.

Mother goes in tomorrow for a "second look" to see if the chemotherapy has been effective. When the original tumor was removed a year ago, cancer cells peppered her small intestines. Dr. Smith will perform a laparoscopy and take tissue samples to biopsy, hoping all is clear. He feels very positive and is looking toward a possible cure.

Mother's strength is returning. She and Dad have been playing tennis again. He tells us her serve is as wicked as ever.

We are all anxious, except Mother. She says it doesn't matter what they find, all we have is now.

CALIFORNIA GULLS

lake level: 4207.75'

"Everything looks good," said Dr. Smith, practically dancing as he entered the room. "All I saw was healthy pink tissue. I couldn't be more pleased."

"So you really think Diane might be clear?" Dad asked. "No more cancer?"

"We won't know for sure until we get the pathology report back on Wednesday, but let's just say, I'm cautiously optimistic. They should be bringing her back to the room any time now. I'll see you on Wednesday."

Dr. Smith left.

Dad and I looked at each other.

"We heard it right? Didn't we?"

"Can you believe it?" I cried. "It's a miracle. I knew Mother could do it. I'll call Steve. Dan and Hank are still in school."

"I'll call the rest of the family," Dad said.

We hurried back to Mother's room to greet her just as the orderlies were wheeling her back. We met her in the hall with thumbs up.

"Honest?" she said a bit drowsy. "Do you promise? Everything was clear?"

Dad and I nodded with tears. She took Dad's hand and wouldn't let it go. At this moment, I realized how badly Mother wanted to live.

She looked at us again. "Really? Everything looked good?"

"Healthy pink tissue," I answer. "Dr. Smith said he couldn't be more pleased."

"I'm almost afraid to believe you—to let myself go," she said. "I just want to sleep, I am so tired. I want to sleep and dream and relax, something I have not allowed myself to do." She took a deep breath, closed her eyes, and sighed. "I can't believe it."

The nurse brought in a bouquet of spring flowers sent by friends.

"Oh, have you ever seen flowers so beautiful?" Mother said. "Bring them closer, please."

Dr. Smith requested that our family meet with him in Mother's room this afternoon. It didn't make sense.

"Why would he want us all here just to reiterate the good news?" Steve asked.

Dad was pacing the halls. "Something's gone wrong," he said. "I can feel it."

Mother was quiet. "I can't believe I was so stupid," she said. "I should never have allowed myself to believe you."

I was sick to my stomach. Dan and Hank sat on the edge of Mother's bed. Brooke leaned against the wall.

Dr. Smith walked into the room with the pathology report.

We all stood. Everyone but Mother. He looked around the room and sat down on an empty chair by the door.

"The pathology report was not as good as I had hoped."

Dad walked out of the room and back in again.

"It's not all bad, but it's not all good either. We found microscopic cells in three of the fifteen biopsies. I'm sorry, Diane, everything looked so good. I was premature in my judgments. It's just that we all wanted it so badly. You've worked so hard and done so well . . ."

Mother shook her head. She was furious. She turned abruptly to Dad and me. "I could have handled this, why couldn't you?"

Dr. Smith tried to continue reassuringly. "There is still a fairly good chance for cure. With six weeks of radiation therapy . . ."

"I don't even want to hear it," Mother said sobbing. "It's over. I'm tired of fighting. Just leave me alone, all of you. Go, please. I need time to myself." She rolled on to her side and faced the wall.

We left. I was heartsick. I had betrayed her. I felt as though I had killed her with my optimism and I was strapped with guilt. Why couldn't I have respected her belief that the outcome mattered less than the gift of each day. We had wanted everything back to its original shape. We had wanted a cure for Mother for ourselves, so we could get on with our lives. What we had forgotten was that she was living hers.

I fled for Bear River, for the birds, wishing someone would rescue me.

The California gulls rescued the Mormons in 1848 from losing their crops to crickets. The gull has become folklore. It is a story we know well.

As word of Great Salt Lake's nasty disposition filtered through the westering grapevine in the 1840's, the appeal of the Great Basin was tainted. The Mormons were an exception. They saw it as Holy Land.

Brigham Young raised his hands above the Salt Lake Valley and said, "This is a good place to make Saints, and it is a good place for Saints to live; it is the place that the Lord has appointed, and we shall stay here until He tells us to go somewhere else."

God's country. Isolation and a landscape of grit were just what the Mormons were looking for. A land that no one else wanted meant religious freedom and community-building without persecution. It was an environment perfectly suited for a people unafraid of what only their hands could yield. They were a people motivated by the dream of Zion. They had found their Dead Sea and the River Jordan. The Great Basin desert was familiar to them if not by sight, at least by story.

But it wasn't easy. Winter quarters for the poorly provisioned families who had just arrived proved difficult. Their livestock had been decimated by wolves and Indian raids. Untended animals grazed down their crops and the harvest of 1847 consisted of only a few "marble-size potatoes." The starving pioneers were reduced to eating "crows, wolf meat, tree bark, thistle tops, sego lily bulbs, and hawks."

One member describes in his journal, "I would dig until I grew weak and faint and sit down and eat a root, and then I would begin again."

The harvest of 1848 looked more promising and the Saints' spirits were buoyed. But just when a full pantry for each family seemed assured, hordes of crickets invaded their wheat fields. The crickets were described as "wingless, dumpy, black, and swollen-headed creatures, with bulging eyes in cases like goggles, mounted upon legs of steel wire . . . a cross between a spider and a buffalo."

The pioneers fought them with brooms, shovels, pitchforks, and fire. Nothing seemed to halt their invasion. In desperation, the farmers and their families fell to their knees with exhaustion and prayed to the Lord for help.

> Upon looking up, I beheld what appeared like a vast flock of pigeons coming from the northwest. It was about three o'clock in the afternoon . . . there must have been thousands of them; their coming was like a great cloud; and when they passed between us and the sun, a shadow covered the field. I could see the gulls settling for more than a mile around us. They were very tame, coming within four or five rods of us.
>
> At first, we thought that they also were after the wheat and this fact added to our terror; but we soon discovered that they devoured only the crickets. Needless to say, we quit fighting and gave our gentle visitors the possession of the fields.

Their prayers had been answered. Their crops had been saved.

Over one hundred years later, Mormons still gather to tell the story of how the gulls freed them from the crickets. How the white angels ate as many crickets as their bellies would hold, flew to the shores of Great Salt Lake and regurgitated them, then returned to the field for more. We honor them as Utah's state bird.

While sitting on the edge of Great Salt Lake, I noticed the gulls flying in one direction. From four o'clock until dusk, with their slow, steady wing beats, they flew southwest. I pocketed this information like a small stone.

The next day, I returned and witnessed the same pilgrimage. After all these years of cohabitation, the gulls had finally, seized my imagination.

I had to follow.

The gulls were flying to their nesting colonies on the islands of Great Salt Lake. What they gain in remoteness (abeyance from predators and human interference) they sacrifice in food supply. Because of its high salinity, Great Salt Lake yields no fish. With the exception of brine shrimp, which make up a meager percentage of the gull's total diet, the water is sterile. Consequently, gulls must fly great distances between island nesting sites and foraging grounds. Round trips between fifty to one hundred miles are made from Hat and Gunnison Islands to the Bear River Migratory Bird Refuge. Daily. White pelicans, double-crested cormorants, and great blue herons, also colony nesters, must make these same migrations to the surrounding marshes of Great Salt Lake.

The population of colony-nesting birds on the islands fluctuates with the lake level and human disturbances. Herons, cormorants, and pelicans are much more sensitive to these pressures than gulls. One striking difference between the species is their territoriality. Herons are wary, skittish. Pelicans and cormorants are shy. If disturbed, great blue herons leave the island first, followed by the pelicans and cormorants. The gulls never leave. They just fly around in circles screaming at the intruders.

The populations of herons, cormorants, and pelicans are decreasing on the islands of Great Salt Lake, whereas evidence shows gull communities on the rise. Gulls are more resilient to change and less vulnerable than other birds to environmental stresses.

William H. Behle, curator of ornithology at the Utah Museum of Natural History, in his classic study on the birds of Great Salt Lake, reported sixty thousand adult California gulls nesting on Gunnison Island on June 29, 1932. This was the highest gull concentration ever known on Great Salt Lake.

Since the flooding, most of the islands have either been abandoned by colony nesters or their populations have been greatly reduced. This seems to have happened for three reasons: lack of nesting space due to rising waters, increased human visitation to the islands, and, most important, lack of food due to the submerged marshes.

In drought conditions, bird populations also decline but for different reasons. In low water, most of the islands are attached to the mainland, making the birds more vulnerable to predators and human interference. Food supply is also threatened as the marshes shrink.

The balance between colony-nesting birds, the fluctuating Great Salt Lake, and its wetlands is a delicate one.

In 1958, Dr. Behle wrote prophetically,

> If present trends continue, there is danger that the islands of Great Salt Lake will be entirely abandoned by colonial birds. Herons already have abandoned all their historic nesting sites on the lake. Cormorants persist at Egg Island but are barely holding their own from year to year. Pelicans faced a critical condition in 1935 and seem to be slowly recovering but their existence is precarious. The gulls are moving to man-made dikes and the islands of the refuges on the east side of the lake.

For now, any remembrance of Great Salt Lake hosting an island archipelago of birds is limited to the journals of early explorers. Captain Howard Stansbury wrote on April 9, 1850,

Rounding the northern point of Antelope Island, we came to a small rocky islet, about a mile west of it, which was destitute of vegetation of any kind, not even a blade of grass being found upon it. It was literally covered with wild waterfowl: ducks, white brandt, blue herons, cormorants, and innumerable flocks of gulls, which had congregated here to build their nests. We found great numbers of these, built of sticks and rushes, in the crevices of the rock, and supplied ourselves without scruple, with as many eggs as we needed, primarily those of the heron, it being too early in the season for most of the other waterfowl.

And on May 8 of the same year:

The neck and shores on both of the little bays were occupied by immense flocks of pelicans and gulls, disturbed now for the first time, probably by the intrusion of man. They literally darkened the air as they rose upon the wing, and hovering over our heads, caused the surrounding rocks to re-echo with their discordant screams. The ground was thickly strewn with their nests, of which there must have been thousands.

I have seen hundreds of gulls nesting not on the islands of Great Salt Lake, but on the old P-dike at the Bear River Migratory Bird Refuge. To wander through a gull colony is disorienting. In the midst of shrieking gulls, you begin to speak, but your voice is silenced. They pull the clouds around you as you walk on eggshells. You quickly realize that you do not belong.

Hundreds of gulls hovered inches above my head, making their shrill repetitive cries, *"Halp! Halp! Halp!"* Several wing tips struck my forehead, a warning that I was too close to their nests. There were so many nests, I didn't know where to step, much less how to behave. Finally, I just stood in one place and watched.

A California gull's nest is a shallow depression on the ground. They gather nesting material and line the hollow. The gull settles down, usually female, and with her body and sometimes the aid of her feet and bill, neatly arranges the feathers, grasses, and twigs into a cup-shaped nest. Depending on the resources available, they can range from simple to elaborate.

The nests at Bear River were simple. Bones from gulls and other animals were woven into their fabric, making them look like death wreathes. Clutches of umber eggs splotched with brown lay in their centers.

Most of the gulls I watched at the Bird Refuge were incubating eggs, an activity which takes from twenty-three to twenty-eight days. Both sexes share in the responsibility.

I wondered in the midst of so many gulls and so many eggs, how the birds could differentiate between them. They do. Parental recognition. The subtle distinctions in patterning and coloration among individual egg clutches test my eye for discrimination. Each brood bears its own coat of arms.

Young gulls are precocial, which means they are relatively well developed at hatching. They are covered with a thick coat of natal down, can leave the nest soon after they hatch, and can feed themselves within a short time. Precocial young are typical to most waterfowl, an adaptation against predators of ground-dwelling birds.

In contrast, altricial young are those birds born helpless, usually naked and with closed eyes, completely dependent on their parents for a sustained period after hatching. Altricial young are more common to passerine birds, which have the advantage of tree nesting. They can afford to be helpless.

It is tempting to pick up a baby gull. I must confess I have tried, but only got as far as its fierce little beak would let me. They come into life as speckled warriors, waving egg teeth on the tips of their upper mandibles. Their battle with the eggshell is tireless as they struggle anywhere from twenty minutes to ten hours. They stand in wet armor ready to face the world.

All around me, eggs were moving, cracking, and breaking open. I would stoop a few feet from a nest and find myself staring eye-to-eye with a chick.

A month from now, in June, the young will be in juvenile plumage, looking like gulls who ventured too close to a campfire. Smoked feathers. They will stretch and beat their wings wildly until one day their own force will surprise them, lifting them a foot or two off the ground. Gradually, with a few running steps, their wings will carry them. In a matter of weeks, adolescent gulls will be agile fliers.

By July, the California gulls will prepare to leave their breeding grounds, taking their young with them. Banding records from Bear River indicate that most of the Great Salt Lake population winters along the Pacific coast from northern Washington to southern California.

I love to watch gulls soar over the Great Basin. It is another trick of the lake to lure gulls inland. On days such as this, when my soul has been wrenched, the simplicity of flight and form above the lake untangles my grief.

"Glide" the gulls write in the sky—and, for a few brief moments, I do.

I go to the lake for a compass reading, to orient myself once again in the midst of change. Each trip is unique. The lake is different. I am different. But the gulls are always here, ordinary—black, white, and gray.

I have refused to believe that Mother will die. And by

denying her cancer, even her death, I deny her life. Denial stops us from listening. I cannot hear what Mother is saying. I can only hear what I want.

But denial lies. It protects us from the potency of a truth we cannot yet bear to accept. It takes our hands and leads us to places of comfort. Denial flourishes in the familiar. It seduces us with our own desires and cleverly constructs walls around us to keep us safe.

I want the walls down. Mother's rage over our inability to face her illness has burned away my defenses. I am left with guilt, guilt I cannot tolerate because it has no courage. I hurt Mother through my own desire to be cured.

I continue to watch the gulls. Their pilgrimage from salt water to fresh becomes my own.

RAVENS

Mother began her radiation treatment this morning. They tattooed her abdomen with black dots and drew a grid over her belly with a blue magic marker.

"After the technicians had turned my body into their bull's-eye," Mother said, "the radiologist casually walked in, read my report, and said, "You realize, Mrs. Tempest, you have less than a 40 percent chance of surviving this cancer.""

"What did you say to him?" I asked as we were driving home.

"I honestly don't remember if I said anything. He rearranged the machinery above me, rearranged my body on the stainless steel slab, and then walked out of the room to zap me and protect himself."

"How do you feel, Mother?" I asked.

She folded her arms across her midriff.

"I feel abused."

This afternoon, I coaxed Mother into going swimming at Great Salt Lake, something we have not done for years. On our backs, we floated, staring up at the sky—the cool water held us—in spite of the light, harsh and blinding. I heard the whisperings of brine shrimp, felt their orange feathered bodies brushing against my own. I showed them to Mother. She shuddered.

We drifted for hours. Merging with salt water and sky so completely, we were resolved, dissolved, in peace.

We returned with salt crystals in our hair and sand in our navels to remind us we had not been dreaming.

The Southern Pacific Railroad Causeway was breached today. Water from the south arm of Great Salt Lake shot through the three-hundred-foot opening into Gunnison Bay like a wave of pent-up emotion.

I envy the release.

Governor Scott Matheson anticipates that the disparate water levels of the south and north arm of Great Salt Lake will equalize within the next couple of months. There will be a mixing of brine as the salt loads within Gunnison and Gilbert Bays redistribute themselves with new bidirectional flow.

A small piece of Great Salt Lake's integrity has been restored.

We celebrated Dad's birthday, July 26, 1933. He reminded Mother, as he does each year, that he is one year younger than she. She retorts each year with the same remark:

"That explains your immaturity and my wisdom." She

reminds him that this year she will be kind to him, that she has not wrapped his presents in black like she did when he turned forty.

Steve, Dan, Hank, and I, together with Brooke and Ann, presented Dad with a large cake flaming with candles.

He is fifty-one.

Great Salt Lake shimmered in the background. It rose another 5' from September 25, 1983, to July 1, 1984, the second-largest rise ever recorded for the lake. The net rise from September 18, 1982 to July 1, 1984 was 9.6'. In comparison, the previously recorded maximum net rise of Great Salt Lake between any two years was 4.7', during 1970 and 1972.

"Make a wish . . ." said Mother. And we watched him blow out the candles.

I wish old Saltair was still standing guard over Great Salt Lake. The magnificent Moorish pavilion built on a wooden trestle reigned supreme during the early 1900s. Its image captures the romance of another era for Utah residents.

Today, I walked where Saltair once stood. A few charred posts from the pier still stand, looking like ravens.

In 1962, Herk Harvey released the film, *Carnival of Souls,* which has become a cult classic, a precursor to *The Night of the Living Dead.* The heroine of the film, Miss Henry, comes to Utah to play the organ. The pastor introduces her to his parish by saying, "We have an organist capable of stirring the soul."

Miss Henry's affinity with the dead leads her in a trance-like journey to Great Salt Lake. As she stands on the boardwalk of Saltair she watches the dead, one after another, emerge from the lake, zombies dripping with salt water. She follows the gaunt, dark-eyed corpses dressed in black into the dance hall, where she is moved to play the organ for them.

For my generation, Saltair had become a sinister piece of abandoned architecture. This was not the case for my grandparents. I recall having dinner with Lettie and Sanky shortly after Saltair had burned to the ground.

My grandfather and grandmother fell in love on moonlit nights at Saltair.

"I remember the way her chiffon dress would blow in the breeze as we stood on the boardwalk looking over the lake. And I remember a kiss or two before we went back inside . . ." he said.

My grandmother smiled as she described the particular peach-colored dress with an asymmetrical hem that she frequently wore to the resort so popular in the 1920s. She boasted about my grandfather's agility at the games of chance, how he would always win a Kewpie doll for her.

They described boarding the open-air train from Salt Lake City to Saltair, how everyone would sing songs in the early evening as the train delivered them to the pavilion perched on wooden trestles above Great Salt Lake.

The dance pavilion catered to some of the great bands of the day: Harry James, Wayne King, Bob Crosby, and Guy Lombardo.

"The dance floor was suspended on springs," my grandmother said. "The ceiling was decorated with huge lighted balls made of mirrors that cast starlight reflections on the dance hall."

"And the band would play until midnight," my grandfather added. "That's when the last train would go back to the city."

Saltair never regained its pre-Depression glamour after it was destroyed by fire the first time on April 12, 1925. Even after it reopened in 1929, the public was becoming more mobile, and the novelty of traveling by train to the lake was beginning to wane. It officially closed in 1968; two years later it was burned down by arsonists.

In 1981, developer Wally Wright, tried to reincarnate Saltair. He purchased a hanger from Hill Air Force Base to use as the structure and then tried to resurrect the Moorish architecture with concrete. It wasn't the same. Somehow, water slides, bumper boats, and fast-food shops didn't hold the integrity of the times. Even so, Wally Wright never got a fair shot at his own concession. Great Salt Lake rose before he completed construction.

And so another abandoned monument to the lake stands. There are ghosts at the Great Salt Lake who still dance on starlit nights.

PINK FLAMINGOS

lake level: 4208.00'

Great Salt Lake has dropped 1.35' during the summer of 1984. About one half of the decline was due to normal evaporation, but the remainder resulted from the breach in the causeway. Perhaps we were given a reprieve.

Mother came over this morning.

"Do you have a minute?" she asked. "Tamra Crocker Pulfer was operated on yesterday for a brain tumor and I want to send her this letter. May I read it to you? I want it to be right."

We walked into the living room. I opened the drapes and we settled on the couch. Mother paused, then began:

> Dearest Tammy:
>
> When I heard of your surgery yesterday, I felt my heart would break. I kept thinking that you are so young to have to go through this. I would gladly, Tammy, take

this cross you are to bear upon my own shoulders if I could. I know what you are going through right now and I want you to know my prayers and love are with you. I wish I could talk to you in person and we could just cry together and share each other's feelings. There are times, however, when you must go through certain things alone and this is one of them. When I say alone, I mean you have to address this illness yourself. You have to decide how you are going to deal with it. I know what a strong young woman you are and what a fighter you can be.

When I was told I had cancer thirteen years ago, I experienced many different reactions. The night before my surgery, I was given a blessing and in the blessing I was told that I would not have cancer, that the lump would be benign, and that I would be fine.

During the surgery, I had a spiritual experience that changed my life. Just before I awakened in the recovery room, I was literally in the arms of my Heavenly Father. I could feel His love for me and how sorry He was that He couldn't keep this from me. What He could and did give me was far greater than not having cancer. He gave me the gifts of faith, hope, strength, love, and a joy and peace I had never felt before. These gifts were my miracle. I know that it is not the trials we are given but how we react to these trials that matters.

I am sending you a book, "The Healing Heart," by Norman Cousins. He has had two incurable illnesses and survived both of them. This book helped me last year more than anything I have ever read. It helped me to realize that I can help in the recuperative process of my own body. That we can help ourselves through positive thinking. In his book, he says, "Death is not the enemy; living in constant fear of it is."

I want to live and think as actively and creatively as it is physically possible for me to do. This year, with two major surgeries, one year of chemotherapy, and six weeks of radiation, has been the most difficult year of my life, and also the most beautiful. It has enabled me to sense and see things I never did before. It brings life into focus one day at a time. You live each moment and when you see the sunset at the end of the day, you are so grateful to be part of that experience.

Don't be so strong, Tammy, that you won't cry when you want to. Let people help you and love you. I can't tell you how important it was for me to let people do things for me. I resisted at first, but I don't know how I would have gotten through the radiation without the six beautiful women who picked me up each day and took me to my treatments. It gave me something to look forward to—each with a different friend—and I appreciated the love and support they gave me.

While I was taking chemotherapy and radiation, I took a lot of vitamins and I believe they helped me stay strong. Let me know if there is anything I can do to help you.

May the Lord bless you, Tammy, with His gifts. You are a very special young woman and I want you to know how much I admire all that you are.

Love, Diane

Mother finished reading the letter. A long silence followed. She looked over to me. "Do you think it's all right to send?"

Our correspondences show us where our intimacies lie. There is something very sensual about a letter. The physical contact of pen to paper, the time set aside to focus thoughts, the folding of the paper into the envelope, licking it closed, addressing it, a chosen stamp, and then the release of the letter to the mailbox—are all acts of tenderness.

And it doesn't stop there. Our correspondences have wings—paper birds that fly from my house to yours— flocks of ideas crisscrossing the country. Once opened, a connection is made. We are not alone in the world.

But how do we correspond with the land when paper and

ink won't do? How do we empathize with the Earth when so much is ravaging her?

The heartbeats I felt in the womb—two heartbeats, at once, my mother's and my own—are heartbeats of the land. All of life drums and beats, at once, sustaining a rhythm audible only to the spirit. I can drum my heartbeat back into the Earth, beating, hearts beating, my hands on the Earth— like a ruffed grouse on a log, beating, hearts beating—like a bittern in the marsh, beating, hearts beating. My hands on the Earth beating, hearts beating. I drum back my return.

"A mirage is created when the air next to the earth becomes warmer than the air immediately above it," said Brooke.

We were walking the salt flats east of Wendover, Nevada, beyond the rock graffiti, where stone signatures have been left in the sand by locals. It was Sunday, mid-September, and hot. A line of quicksilver danced ahead of us.

"I don't believe it's a mirage," I said. "It looks like another finger of Great Salt Lake."

"It's a mirage, Ter," Brooke continued. "The lake we are seeing is actually the sand's surface appearing wet, due to the hot air immediately above it and the cooler air above that. See how we are standing on slightly higher ground looking down?"

"So?"

"So, as a result of bending light rays, the image of the sky is turned upside down. It just looks like a lake."

"I think it is the lake."

We keep walking toward it, to prove ourselves right. But the body of water that I see and Brooke distrusts keeps flowing farther away from us. We retreat and the lake seems to follow.

I concede.

Brooke grins. I forget he is a biologist with an analytic mind.

"It's all an illusion. Nothing is as it appears. The air refracting the sun's rays, transforming sand into water; make sense?"

I look at him and nod. "I think it's about hope on a hot day."

Mother and Dad are in Switzerland. I received a letter from her today. It reads:

Dear Terry:

More and more, I am realizing the natural world is my connection to myself. Landscape brings me simplicity. I can shed the multiplicity of things at home and take one duffle bag wherever I go. How wonderful to shed clothes and be free of choices, to feel the sun on my back and the wind on my face. I find my peace, my solitude, in the time I am alone in nature.

John has been my guide, Terry. His nature is not to just sit back and be an observer to the land, but an active participant. When we went to Hawaii for the first time, nineteen years ago, we ran and embraced it all. We didn't just look at the ocean, we dove into the waves and tasted salt water on our lips. We greeted the sunrise on the crater in Maui and looked out over thousands of miles. I'll swear we saw the curvature of the earth. We celebrated each day by walking along the beach, picking up shells. We ran into the wind and fell on to the sand, watching the tiny sandpipers dart back and forth.

And we are doing that now. We are hiking up and down the Alps together, walking farther than I ever thought possible. We have slept on the grass next to cows with bells around their necks. We have walked thigh-high in wildflowers. The natural world is a third party in our marriage. It holds us close and lets us revel in the intimacy of all that is real.

I think of you constantly. Please give our love to everyone at home.

We love you,
Mother

I fold the letter back into its envelope and call Brooke. Perhaps, we can go south this weekend.

I love to make lists. Maybe it's my background in beehives and breadmaking, the whole business of being industrious and frugal (of which I am neither) that a list promotes. Or maybe it's the power that comes when you can cross something off a list. Done. Finished. Move on to the next chore. I can see in a very tangible form what I have accomplished in a day. Or perhaps it's the democratic nature of lists that I find so attractive. Each task is of equal importance on paper. So "pick up fresh flowers" carries the same weight as "do the laundry." It's the line slashed through the words that counts. Never mind that the pleasurable items are crossed off by noon and the difficult ones, meant for procrastination anyway, get moved to the next day's agenda. The point is that my intentions are honorable. My lists will defend me.

The life list of a birdwatcher is of a different order. It's not what you cross off that counts, but what you add. It is a tally of all the species of birds seen within a lifetime. A bird seen for the first time is called "a lifer."

The life list can be a private accounting of birds seen, a scrapbook of sorts, of places visited and birds watched. It provides the pleasure of traditional list-making (in this case, adding something new to the list instead of crossing something off). Those who use their bird list in this manner usually have no idea of their total sum of species. And it is done at random—when a person thinks about it.

At the end of each day, I write down the names of all birds seen and read them out loud, regardless of who is there. It's like throwing a party and afterwards talking about who came. There are always those you can count on and those who will surprise you. And, once in a blue moon, an accidental guest will arrive.

Within every checklist there are those birds listed as "accidentals," one species, or at best a few, that have wandered far from their normal range. They are flukes in a flock of predictable migrants. They are loners in an unfamiliar territory.

William H. Behle, author of *Utah Birds,* defines an accidental as "a species seen only one or two times since 1920 or one or two times in the last fifty years or another fifty year interval provided that species is just as likely to occur now as then." Accidental birds in Utah are substantiated by at least one recorded specimen.

On July 25, 1962, Don Neilson, manager of the Clear Lake Refuge, observed an American flamingo in Millard County, Utah. It stayed in the area through Columbus Day. He has color photographs to prove it.

Another sighting occurred on August 3, 1966, by W. E. Ritter and Reuben Dietz who saw a flamingo at Buffalo Bay, on the northeast shore of Antelope Island. The bird was washed out and pale, thousands of miles from its homeland, so they inferred it must be an escapee from Tracy Aviary or Hogle Zoo in Salt Lake City. Calls were made, but all captive flamingos were accounted for.

Then, in the summer of 1971, a third flamingo was seen at the Bear River Migratory Bird Refuge from early June through September 29. Once again, photographs verified the sighting.

I personally have seen flamingos throughout the state of Utah perched proudly on lawns and in the gravel gardens of trailer courts. These flamingos, of course, are not *Phoenicopterus ruber,* but pink, plastic flamingos that can easily be purchased at any hardware store.

It is curious that we need to create an environment foreign from our own. In 1985, over 450,000 plastic flamingos were purchased in the United States. And the number is rising.

Pink flamingos teetering on suburban lawns—our unnatural link to the natural world.

The flocks of flamingos that Louis Agassiz Fuertes lovingly painted in the American tropics are no longer accessible to us. We have lost the imagination to place them in a dignified world. And when they do grace the landscapes around us, they are considered "accidental." We no longer believe in the possibility of such things.

There have been other accidentals in Utah.

On July 2, 1919, a flock of five roseate spoonbills flew over the Barnes Ranch near Wendover, Nevada. Mr. Barnes, having never seen such a bird, shot one and kept it inside his house for years as a conversation piece. It strangely disappeared and was subsequently found; it now rests at the Utah Museum of Natural History.

The flamingo and roseate spoonbill are not the only rarities to visit the wetlands surrounding Great Salt Lake. Other accidentals include the European wigeon seen at the Bear River Bird Refuge on October 19, 1955, and another one sighted by Bill Pingree at the Lakefront Gun Club on December 15, 1963.

And when there is a species whose occurrence is open to question largely by virtue of the absence of a record specimen (a bird in the hand), but where the competence of the observer or observers constitutes "sufficient evidence to justify the inclusion of the species in the checklist," these birds are listed as "hypothetical." Hypothetical species sighted around Great Salt Lake include the red-necked grebe, reddish egret, Louisiana heron, harlequin duck, black scoter, black oystercatcher, wandering tattler, stilt sandpiper, bar-tailed godwit, parakeet auklet, northern parula warbler, and a palm warbler.

How can hope be denied when there is always the possibility of an American flamingo or a roseate spoonbill floating down from the sky like pink rose petals?

How can we rely solely on the statistical evidence and percentages that would shackle our lives when red-necked grebes, bar-tailed godwits, and wandering tattlers come into our country?

When Emily Dickinson writes, "Hope is the thing with feathers that perches in the soul," she reminds us, as the birds do, of the liberation and pragmatism of belief.

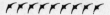

SNOW BUNTINGS

lake level: 4209.15'

The eastern shore of Great Salt Lake is frozen, and for as far as I can see it translates into isolation. Desolation. The fog hangs low, with little delineation between earth and sky. A few ravens. A few eagles. And the implacable wind.

Snow crystals stand on the land like the raised hackles of wolves. Broken reeds and cattails are encased in ice. Great Salt Lake has not only entered the marsh, it has taken over.

Because of the high water level and the drop in salinity, Great Salt Lake can freeze and does. The transparent ice along the lake's edge is filled with bubbles of air trapped inside like the sustained notes of a soprano.

I walk these open spaces in silence, relishing the monotony of the Refuge in winter.

Perhaps I am here because of last night's dream, when I stood on the frozen lake before a kayak made of sealskin.

I walked on the ice toward the boat and picked up a handful of shredded hide and guts. An old Eskimo man said, "You have much to work with." Suddenly, the kayak was stripped of its skin. It was a rib cage of willow. It was the skeleton of a fish.

I want to see it for myself, wild exposure, in January, when this desert is most severe. The lake is like steel. I wrap my alpaca shawl tight around my face until only my eyes are exposed. I must keep walking to stay warm. Even the land is frozen. There is no give beneath my feet.

I want to see the lake as Woman, as myself, in her refusal to be tamed. The State of Utah may try to dike her, divert her waters, build roads across her shores, but ultimately, it won't matter. She will survive us. I recognize her as a wilderness, raw and self-defined. Great Salt Lake strips me of contrivances and conditioning, saying, "I am not what you see. Question me. Stand by your own impressions."

We are taught not to trust our own experiences. Great Salt Lake teaches me experience is all we have.

One month ago, this was frozen country, mono-chromatic and still. This morning, spring has moved in. Constellations of ducks: pintails, mallards, wigeons, and teals are flying in from the south and southwest. The air is wild with voices, avian dialects are being spoken from every direction. The sky vibrates with wings.

Mother does not share my affection for birds. This is her first trip to Bear River. We watch a dozen herons fishing. Beyond them, I spot a carcass, a scattering of blue feathers and bones. I lure Mother forward. Up ahead, we find a wing.

"A great blue heron . . ." I say, picking it up. The primary feathers are attached to the ulna like the teeth of a comb.

Blood stains the snow. More bones. More feathers. And tracks.

We bend down to get a closer look.

"What do you think?" asks Mother.

"Fox, maybe. I don't know. I think they're too small for a coyote."

The wind blows, scattering the white, downy feathers in all directions. They rest momentarily on the snow, rocking back and forth like cradles, until they cartwheel off in the breeze.

We walk west. Blue-winged teals congregate between greasewood. On the road adjacent to Great Salt Lake, huge compression fractures have heaved diagonal chunks of ice this way and that. I try to climb over them, but they present too great an obstacle. They line the shore for miles. We can travel no farther.

"I want you to read 'God Sees the Truth, but Waits,'" said Mother. "Tolstoy writes about a man, wrongly accused of a murder, who spends the rest of his life in a prison camp. Twenty-six years later, as a convict in Siberia, he meets the true murderer and has an opportunity to free himself, but chooses not to. His longing for home leaves him and he dies."

I ask Mother why this story matters to her.

"Each of us must face our own Siberia," she says. "We must come to peace within our own isolation. No one can rescue us. My cancer is my Siberia."

Suddenly, two white birds about the size of finches, dart in front of us and land on the snow.

"I don't know these birds, Mother. They're something new."

She hands me the bird book. I rapidly thumb through the pages. She is looking through the binoculars.

"They are white with black on their backs and I see a flash

of rust on their heads." She pauses, "I can also see black on the tips of their wings when they fly . . ."

I quickly look up to see if they are gone, but they have just moved a few feet up the road. I flip back through the book again.

"I found them! Here they are—page 412, snow buntings!" I hand the field guide to Mother, focusing on the birds to make sure.

"I can't believe it!" I look at her, then back to the buntings. "These are rare to the Refuge. I've never seen them before."

We watch them forage around the edges of melting snow. Mother brings down her binoculars.

"Where are they usually found?" she asks, looking at the field guide once again, this time at the map illustrating bunting distribution.

"Snow buntings are circumpolar, nesting in the Arctic on the tundra."

Mother watches the birds carefully. "Tell me, Terry, are these birds Tolstoy may have known?"

Mother and I met for lunch today. She shared with me the letter she received from Tamra Crocker Pulfer. It read:

Dear Diane:

I feel you understand maybe far more than I do about this difficult time. The letter you sent was so good for me, and your constant support of myself and my mother have been deeply needed.

I've learned a most valuable lesson. Sometimes you have to totally rely on the arms, tears, and loving hearts of others, that this is truly where God's love lies, in the support of family and friends.

I appreciate the book you sent me and the lotion for

my twenty-ninth birthday. I really thought I would go gray before I went bald.

I wish at times, I had more options and choices. But right now, I am torn between the excitement of what I am learning about life and the sorrow I feel in that I have no future.

My beliefs are carrying me, Diane. How exciting to know that we will possibly be able to design and create our own worlds as our Father and Mother in Heaven have.

I am starting to forget days now, and often around 4:00 a.m., my pillow becomes wet with the challenges ahead. I am crying, Diane. Please, I say, help me laugh and mean it, help me find gratitude for the small things I have left.

Diane, never before have I wanted to do more, but I can't concentrate on what it is that I want. And then when I remember, I don't have the strength or the energy to carry it out. I know I want Adrian, Canace, Christian, Jeneva, and mostly, just to nurse and hold sweet Adrea. How can we be so sad and so full at the same time?

I say to myself, be cheerful and don't worry about the future. But then I think about my children. I wish I could interview one hundred robust women who had hearts of gold, to raise my family and teach them what I have taught them. Maybe next week, I'll place an ad in the newspaper.

Thank you for your example, Diane. I will love you forever.

Tamra

The eye of the cormorant is emerald. The eye of the eagle is amber. The eye of the grebe is ruby. The eye of the ibis is sapphire. Four gemstones mirror the minds of birds, birds who mediate between heaven and earth.

We miss the eyes of birds, focusing only on feathers.

WHITE PELICANS

lake level: 4209.90'

The Refuge is subdued, unusually quiet. The spring frenzy of courtship and nesting is absent, because there is little food and habitat available. Although the species count remains about the same, individual numbers are down. Way down. This afternoon, I watched a white-faced ibis nest float alongside a drowned cottonwood tree. Three eggs had been abandoned. I did not see the adults.

A colony-nesting bird survey has been initiated this spring by the Utah Division of Wildlife Resources to monitor changes in population and habitat use of selected species affected by the rising Great Salt Lake.

The historical nesting grounds on the islands of Great Salt Lake are gone, with the exception of a California gull colony on Antelope Island and the white pelicans on Gunnison. This means colony nesters are now dependent upon the vegetation surrounding the lake for their livelihood.

Great blue herons, snowy egrets, cattle egrets, and double-crested cormorants use trees, tall shrubs, or man-made structures for nesting.

Franklin gulls, black-crowned night herons, and white-faced ibises nest in emergent vegetation such as bulrushes and cattails.

American avocets, black-necked stilts, and other shorebirds are ground nesters who usually scrape together a few sticks around clumps of low-lying vegetation such as salt grass and pickleweed.

Don Paul, waterfowl biologist for the Division of Wildlife Resources, anticipates that the white-faced ibis and Franklin gull populations will be the hardest hit by the flood.

"Look around and tell me how many stands of bulrush you see?" He waves his hand over the Refuge. "It's gone, and I suspect, so are they. We should have our data compiled by the end of the summer."

I turn around three hundred and sixty degrees: water as far as I can see. The echo of Lake Bonneville lapping against the mountains returns.

The birds of Bear River have been displaced; so have I.

Nothing is familiar to me any more. I just returned home from the hospital, having had a small cyst removed from my right breast. Second time. It was benign. But I suffered the uncertainty of not knowing for days. My scars portend my lineage. I look at Mother and I see myself. Is cancer my path, too?

As a child, I was aware that my grandmother, Lettie, had only one breast. It was not a shocking sight. It was her body. She loved to soak in steaming, hot baths, and I would sit beside the tub and read her my favorite fairy tales.

"One more," she would say, completely relaxed. "You read so well."

What I remember is my grandmother's beauty—her moist, translucent skin, the way her body responded to the slow squeeze of her sponge, which sent hot water trickling over her shoulders. And I loved how she smelled like lavender.

Seeing Mother's scar did not surprise me either. It was not radical like her mother's. Her skin was stretched smooth and taut across her chest, with the muscles intact.

"It is an inconvenience," Mother said. "That's all."

When I look in the mirror and Brooke stands behind me and kisses my neck, I whisper in his ear, "Hold my breasts."

Hundreds of white pelicans stand shoulder to shoulder on an asphalt spit that eventually disappears into Great Salt Lake. They do not look displaced as they engage in head-bobbing, bill-snapping, and panting; their large, orange gular sacs fanning back and forth act as a cooling device. Some preen. Some pump their wings. Others stand, take a few steps forward, tip their bodies down, and then slide into the water, popping up like corks. Their immaculate white forms with carrotlike bills render them surreal in a desert landscape.

Home to the American white pelicans of Great Salt Lake is Gunnison Island, one hundred sixty-four acres of bare-boned terrain. Located in the northwest arm of the lake, it is nearly one mile long and a half-mile wide, rising approximately two hundred seventy-eight feet above the water.

So far, the flooding of Great Salt Lake has favored pelicans. The railroad trestle connecting the southern tip of the Promontory peninsula with the eastern shore of the lake slowed the rate of salt water intrusion into Bear River Bay.

The high levels of stream inflow help to keep much of Bear River Bay fresh, so fish populations are flourishing. So are the pelicans.

Like the California gulls, the pelicans of Gunnison Island must make daily pilgrimages to freshwater sites to forage on carp or chub. Many pelican colonies fly by day and forage by night, to take advantage of desert thermals. The isolation of Gunnison Island offers protection to young pelicans, because there are no predators aside from heat and relentless gulls. Bear River Bay remains their only feeding site on Great Salt Lake.

So are their social skills. White pelicans are gregarious. What one does, they all do. Take fishing for example: four, five, six, as many as a dozen or more forage as a group, forming a circle to corral and then to herd fish, almost like a cattle drive, toward shallower water where they can more efficiently scoop them up in their pouches.

Cooperative fishing has advantages. It concentrates their food source, conserves their energy, and yields results: the pelicans eat. They return to Gunnison Island with fish in their bellies (not in their pouches) and invite their young to reach deep inside their throats as they regurgitate morsels of fish.

It's not a bad model, cooperation in the name of community. Brigham Young tried it. He called it the United Order.

The United Order was a heavenly scheme for a totally self-sufficient society based on the framework of the Mormon Church. It was a seed of socialism planted by a conservative people. So committed was this "American Moses" to the local production of every needful thing that he even initiated a silkworm industry to wean the Saints from their dependence on the Orient for fine cloth.

Brigham Young, the pragmatist, received his inspiration

for the United Order not so much from God as from Lorenzo Snow, a Mormon apostle, who in 1864 established a mercantile cooperative in the northern Utah community named after the prophet. Brigham City became the model of people working on behalf of one another.

The town, situated on Box Elder Creek at the base of the Wasatch Mountains, sixty miles north of Salt Lake City, was founded in 1851. It consisted of some six families until 1854, when Lorenzo Snow moved to Brigham City with fifty additional families. He had been called by Brother Brigham to settle there and preside over the Latter-day Saints in that region.

The families that settled Brigham City were carefully chosen by the church leadership. Members included a schoolteacher, a mason, carpenter, blacksmith, shoemaker, and other skilled craftsmen and tradesmen who would ensure the economic and social vitality of the community.

Lorenzo Snow was creating a community based on an ecological model: cooperation among individuals within a set of defined interactions. Each person was operating within their own "ecological niche," strengthening and sustaining the overall structure or "ecosystem."

Apostle Snow, with a population of almost sixteen hundred inhabitants to provide for, organized a cooperative general store. Mormon historian Leonard J. Arrington explains, "It was his intention to use this mercantile cooperative as the basis for the organization of the entire economic life of the community and the development of the industries needed to make the community self-sufficient."

A tannery, a dairy, a woolen factory, sheep herds, and hogs were added to the Brigham City Cooperative. Other enterprises included a tin shop, rope factory, cooperage, greenhouse and nursery, brush factory, and a wagon and carriage repair shop. An education department supervised the school and seminary.

The community even made provisions for transients, declaring a "tramp department" which enlisted their labor for chopping wood in exchange for a good meal.

After the Brigham City Cooperative was incorporated into Brigham Young's United Order, members were told,

> If brethren should be so unfortunate as to have any of their property destroyed by fire, or otherwise, the United Order will rebuild or replace such property for them. When these brethren, or any other members of the United Order die, the directors become the guardians of the family, caring for the interests and inheritances of the deceased for the benefit and maintenance of the wives and children, and when the sons are married, giving them a house and stewardship, as the father would have done for them. Like care will be taken of their interests if they are sent on missions or taken sick.

By 1874, the entire economic life of this community of four hundred families was owned and directed by the cooperative association. There was no other store in town. Fifteen departments (later to expand to forty) produced the goods and services needed by the community; each household obtained its food, clothing, furniture, and other necessities from these sources.

In 1877, the secretary of the association filed the total capital stock as $191,000 held among 585 shareholders. The total income paid by the various departments to some 340 employees was in excess of $260,000.

Brigham Young's ideal society where "all members would be tending to their own specialty" appeared to be in full bloom. The Brigham City Cooperative even caught the eye of British social reformer Brontier O'Brien. He noted that the Mormons had "created a soul under the ribs of death." Edward Bellamy spent a week in Brigham City researching *Looking Backward,* a Utopian novel prophesying a new social and economic order.

Home industry was proving to be solid economics.

But signs of inevitable decay began to show. A descendant of a Brigham City man told Arrington that his grandfather formed a partnership with another prominent Brigham City citizen in the late 1860s. Their haberdashery was the only place in town where material other than homespun could be purchased. When they succeeded beyond their dreams, they were asked to join the association. They declined, and townfolk were immediately instructed not to trade with them. When some of the community persisted in trading with these men, despite orders from Church officials, members of the Church were placed at the door of the shop to record the names of all persons who did business inside, even though the men in partnership were Mormons in good standing. As a result of this tactic, the business soon failed and the men were forced to set up shop elsewhere.

The ecological model of the Brigham City Cooperative began to crumble. They were forgetting one critical component: diversity.

The United Order of Minutes, taken on July 20, 1880, states, "It was moved and carried unanimously that the council disapprove discountenance, and disfellowship all persons who would start an opposition store or who would assist to erect a building for that purpose."

History has shown us that exclusivity in the name of empire building eventually fails. Fear of discord undermines creativity. And creativity lies at the heart of adaptive evolution.

Lorenzo Snow's fears that the Brigham City Cooperative would not adapt and respond quickly enough to the needs of a growing population materialized. Fire, debt, taxes, and fines befell the Order. In 1885, Apostle Snow was indicted on a charge of unlawful cohabitation (polygamy). He served eleven months in the Utah State Penitentiary before his conviction was set aside by the United States Supreme Court. Finally, as a result of the 1890s depression, the cooperative store went bankrupt. By 1896, all that remained of Brigham City's hive of industry was the unused honey stored on the shelves of the new general store.

Fifteen years of United Order graced Brigham City, Utah. A model for community cooperation? In part. But there is an organic difference between a system of self-sufficiency and a self-sustaining system. One precludes diversity, the other necessitates it. Brigham Young's United Order wanted to be independent from the outside world. The Infinite Order of Pelicans suggests there is no such thing.

"Can you count?" Don Paul asks me one morning at the Ogden airport.

"1, 2, 3 . . ." I joke.

"Get in, you'll do fine."

We board *Skywagon II* for Gunnison Island for the Division of Wildlife Resources annual count of breeding pelicans.

We are cleared and begin taxiing down the runway. In a few seconds we are airborne, flying over farmlands. The checkerboards of crops, so familiar to rural communities become submerged and suddenly, we are flying over water. To see how much Great Salt Lake dominates the landscape from the air is to adopt a radical respect for its geography.

"I had no idea . . ." I mused.

"Nobody does," answers Don. "Except for the birds."

Images of the Utah poet, Alfred Lambourne come to mind as we look out over his "inland sea."

> In outline the sea is peculiar, resembling somewhat a human hand. The fingers are pressed together and point north, northwest. The stretch of water forming the thumb is known as Bear River Bay, and the dividing mountains between thumb and fingers is Promontory Range. In the palm of the hand are four large islands— Stansbury, Antelope, Carrington, and Fremont. Three which are smaller lie away to the north—Strong's Knob, Gunnison, and Dolphin.

While Lorenzo Snow was maintaining the United Order, Lambourne was living out his own order of solitude on Gunnison Island. Lambourne inhabited the island for one year in 1895, with the hope of homesteading seventy-five acres. But his application was denied, the rationale being that the island was more suitable for mineral interests than agriculture. Given the Mormon Church's religious doctrine against the drinking of alcohol, his carefully tended vineyard did not do much to bolster his request for residency.

I can see the flooded offices of the Bear River Migratory Bird Refuge on my right. Herons and cormorants are nesting on the roofs. Fremont Island, on our left, looks like a piece of worked flint.

"No colony nesters down there," says Paul. "No native grasses. No nothing. Only Welsh ponies and sheep. That island has been beaten to death. It's privately owned now. Kit Carson painted a cross on one of those rock outcrops, but darned if I can find it. I've tried."

The pilot, Val, banks the plane to the left. Three more islands come into view.

"There's Stansbury, Carrington, and the tiny island beyond is Hat, formerly known as Bird Island. It used to be covered with nesting pelicans, herons, gulls, terns, and cormorants. As you can see now, it's almost underwater."

Below us, rust ribbons of brine oscillate with the currents. Gulls, grebes, and phalaropes feed along the shrimp lines.

"There's practically no brine left in the south arm," Paul says. "As a result, most of the phalaropes and grebes have moved up here."

"Up ahead, Gunnison Island," the pilot reports. Lambourne's description is accurate:

> It is a rock, a rising of the partially submerged Desert Range of mountains, a summit of black limestone with longitudinal traversements of coarse conglomerates.

The plane circles the island rounding the west shore. The pilot banks hard to the right so Don Paul can get a solid counting. He begins charting the nesting pelicans. The island is beaded with them.

"Most of these birds are young," He explains. "The adults are feeding at Bear River Bay. I saw them feeding as we flew over."

We circle the island once again, while he continues counting, marking dots on his map of Gunnison.

"The colonies look like they're all synchros."

"Synchros?" I ask.

The plane crosses over to the east shore, which appears rockier. I see no pelicans nesting on this side.

"The reproductive activities of pelicans within a specific colony are highly synchronized. Egg-laying, hatching, and fledging of chicks in any given colony usually occurs within a five- to nine-day period."

We swing around the west shore of the island. He asks Val to bank right again and fly as low as he can.

"But the interesting part of this environmental story is that the reproductive activities of the pelican population on Gunnison Island as a whole is asynchronous. The reproductive-cycle stages between colonies may differ by as much as four to eight weeks."

"What's the advantage?" I ask.

"Scientists hypothesize that coloniality increases an individual's chance of successfully finding food, either by an exchange of information within a colony about where food is particularly abundant, or by enabling pelicans to form groups, leaving the island in flocks so they can take advantage of the thermals. Then, when they find their foraging grounds, they will fish cooperatively."

"Colonial economics," Don Paul continues, "would not be advantageous if every colony was on the same breeding and feeding schedule. The competition for food would not only diminish the resource but also result in pelican mortality. Whereas, a month later, it's a different ballgame: there's plenty of food to go around. The staggering of intercolony development on Gunnison Island makes good ecological sense."

"We'll catch them one more time," says Val. "There's the triangulation post set up by Stansbury in 1850."

I can see three sticks on top of one of the peaks. I try to locate Lambourne's cabin but can only find the guano miner's shack. As we circle the island for the last time, I recognize the northern cliffs, which Lambourne describes as "a conchant lion. His massive head turned eastward, his monstrous paws rest on the lower shelves."

Not much has changed.

"That's it . . ." says Paul as *Skywagon II* levels and straightens for home.

"And the count?" I ask.

Don Paul looks over his papers. "Ten thousand breeding adults."

Water. Rock. Bird. I don't know if Brigham Young ever ventured to Gunnison Island or observed the finely tuned society of pelicans. But had his attention been focused more on Earth than "heaven on earth" his vision for managing the Saints in the Great Basin might have been altered.

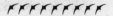

YELLOW=HEADED
BLACKBIRDS

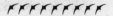

lake level: 4209.55'

Mother's health seems to be stable.

Great Salt Lake seems to be stable. I've waited a long time to see Fish Springs National Wildlife Refuge. Now seems to be a good time. It is another oasis in the desert, adjacent to the Desert Test Center, one of the many military bombing ranges in the Great Basin.

I follow the old Pony Express Trail through miles of sagebrush. It's a four-hour drive west from Salt Lake City. Eye-squinting country. A thin green line appears on the horizon. Bulrushes. The liquid, lambent stage for birds.

They are all here: avocets, stilts, waterfowl galore, great blues, night herons, bitterns and blackbirds, willets, ibises, marsh hawks, and terns. I sit on the edge of the springs, my eyes unable to focus, as a black-and-white-winged dragonfly is snapped by the mandibles of a snowy egret.

Dusk is approaching. Meadowlarks and yellow-headed

blackbirds sing the shadows longer. Lake Bonneville has left its mark. Bathtub rings rim the Great Basin. Tonight these mountains are lavender with blue creases that fall like chintz.

First stars appear. A crescent moon. I throw down my sleeping bag. The stillness of the desert instructs me like a trail of light over water.

There are dunes beyond Fish Springs. Secrets hidden from interstate travelers. They are the armatures of animals. Wind swirls around the sand and ribs appear. There is musculature in dunes.

And they are female. Sensuous curves—the small of a woman's back. Breasts. Buttocks. Hips and pelvis. They are the natural shapes of Earth. Let me lie naked and disappear. Crypsis.

The wind rolls over me. Particles of sand skitter across my skin, fill my ears and nose. I am aware only of breathing. The workings of my lungs are amplified. The wind picks up. I hold my breath. It massages me. A raven lands inches away. I exhale. The raven flies.

Things happen quickly in the desert.

REDHEADS

lake level: 4208.50'

September, 1985. Don Paul's study is out. The recent population and habitat studies performed by the Utah Division of Wildlife Resources shows that colony nesting species around Great Salt Lake have been affected by the rise in lake level. Some are adapting and some are not. The data collection was funded by Los Angeles City Power and Light, which was recently sued by the National Wildlife Federation for drawing down the water levels of Mono Lake.

Great blue herons, egrets, and cormorants, all tree nesters, have been aided by the flooding of the wetlands, as waterfowl management areas have become inaccessible to man and arboreal predators. Their preferred habitat for nesting: dead trees. Suddenly, there's lots of them, killed by the rising salt water. The cottonwoods and box elders that once provided shade and cover for songbirds have become bare-branched rookeries for herons and cormorants.

They have not been without their problems, however. In some instances, where they had used the low tamarisk shrubs to nest in, eggs and young were drowned as the waters rose over a few weeks.

As was expected, white-faced ibises and Franklin gulls, both dependent on hard-stem bulrushes for nesting, have suffered the most. With 80 percent of the world's population of white-faced ibises nesting in Utah, these losses become significant.

In 1979, the Utah ibis population was estimated at 8690 pairs. The 1985 colony-nesting survey recorded 3438 pairs. The decline in Franklin gulls is even more radical: a late 1970s survey showed a thousand breeding pairs, compared to the fifty-one nests counted this year.

It is hoped that many breeding adult ibises and Franklin gulls have survived and moved on to more stable marshes in the Great Basin. Breeding numbers are reported higher at Fish Springs and at the Ruby Marshes in Nevada. The Cutler and Bear Lake marshes northeast of Bear River also show an increase in ibis and gull populations.

The avocets and stilts, along with other ground nesters around Great Salt Lake, have been completely displaced. Their nesting sites have been usurped by water, with mudflats almost nonexistent. Some pairs of avocets have been seen nesting just off the interstate on gravel shoulders.

California has lost 95 percent of its wetlands over the past one hundred years. Eighty-five percent of Utah's wetlands have been lost in the last two. When wetlands are destroyed, many species go with them, and not just the birds that nest there. In Utah's case, tiger salamanders, leopard frogs, orchids, buttercups, myriads of insects and rodents, plus the birds and mammals that prey on them, are vanishing.

Marshes are among the most productive ecosystems on the planet. They are also among the most threatened.

Nationwide, seventy-six endangered species are dependent upon wetlands. Marshes all across the country are disappearing without fanfare, leaving the earth devoid of birdsong. The long-billed curlews who lose their broods to floods become a generation that much more precious to their species' survival. Whether it's because of drought, as is the case in the prairie pothole region to the north, or levels of high toxicity in California's central valley, or just plain development—our wetlands are disappearing.

Wetlands are one more paradox of Great Salt Lake. The marshes here are disappearing naturally. It's not the harsh winter or yearly spillover that threatens Utah's wetland birds and animals. It is lack of land. In the normal cycle of a rising Great Salt Lake, the birds would simply move up. New habitat would be found. New habitat would be created. They don't have those options today, as they find themselves flush against freeways and a rapidly expanding airport.

Refugees.

Before the rise of Great Salt Lake, thousands of whistling swans (now called "tundra swans" by the American Ornithologists' Union) descended on Bear River Bay each autumn. As many as sixty thousand swans have been counted at the Bear River Migratory Bird Refuge during mid-October and mid-November, making it the single largest concentration of migrating swans in North America.

In November 1984, only two hundred fifty-nine whistling swans were counted at the Refuge. One year later: three.

Birds are opportunistic by nature, but resourcefulness fails in the presence of high-speed traffic and asphalt.

This year, the Utah State Legislature appropriated $98

million for flood control. The alternatives state waterfowl managers are reviewing are: wait for the lake to recede, as it inevitably will; try to acquire more habitat, especially newly created wetlands; or reduce the level of the lake.

Tim Provan, the waterfowl biologist for the Division of Wildlife Resources in Salt Lake City, points out that "The marshes don't produce young. They never have. They hold the birds during migration. The marshes let them rest and feed for extended periods—two, three, four months at a time. The seven to eight hundred thousand ducks we did produce have dropped 85 percent since the flood."

He goes on to say, "The Great Salt Lake marshes had one of the strongest populations of redheads, but they are extremely susceptible to high water. They have been hit the hardest. They are not producing young. Their population is down 60 to 80 percent. We have found a direct statistical relationship between loss of habitat and rate of production: 70 percent loss of habitat, 70 percent loss of young. Our redheads are going other places where they are less successful breeders and more subject to predation." He stares out his office window. "I've seen redheads, canvasbacks, shovelers, and teals just lying dormant in the water as though they were in shock."

"How long before the marshes of Bear River will return?" I ask him.

"It will be three to seven years after the lake recedes before it even begins to take a significant turn, because the soil is so saturated with salts. The recycling of nutrients, the reseeding of plants—that will be a fifteen- to twenty-year turnaround."

"The truth is, the system isn't out there to replace. No other system on the continent can replace or absorb this wetland complex. There is a certain threshold that once crossed, we can never recover. When the death rates exceed the birth rates, we are in trouble. Nobody knows the answers. We are working with the questions."

KILLDEER

lake level: 4208.40'

Mimi and Mother and I had our astrology done. It seemed like a reasonable thing to do. As Mimi said, "If it sheds light on all the confusion, why not?"

We decided to have a picnic by Great Salt Lake to discuss our charts. We sat on its edge where large boulders had been brought in to secure the shore. Each of us found our own niche in the sun. Three women: a Leo, a Pisces, a Virgo. A grandmother, mother, and daughter.

It was beautiful and it was hot. We saw six ruddy ducks, one pair of redheads, avocets and stilts, flocks of Franklin gulls, young shrikes on greasewood, and meadowlarks.

Mimi and I engaged in our birding ritual: locate, focus, observe, and identify. After the bird flies, we pore over the field guide and debate over which species we have just seen.

Mother was amused, saying she wished she liked birds as much as we did, but she had never recovered from Alfred

Hitchcock's film "The Birds." She could see herself all too well as Tippi Hedren fleeing from the wrath of gulls, regardless of whether they were ring-billed or California.

"So what do you believe?" Mother asked.

"I believe every woman should own at least one pair of red shoes . . ." I answered.

Mother grinned, "I'm being serious."

"So am I."

"When I was a young woman with four children, I was always living ahead of myself," she said. "Everything I was doing was projected toward the future, and I was so busy, busy, busy, preparing for tomorrow, for the next week, for the next month. Then one day, it all changed. At thirty-eight years old, I found I had breast cancer. I can remember asking my doctor what I should plan for in my future. He said, 'Diane, my advice to you is to live each day as richly as you can.' As I lay in my bed after he left, I thought, will I be alive next year to take my son to first grade? Will I see my children marry? And will I know the joy of holding my grandchildren?" She looked out over the water, barefoot, her legs outstretched; a white visor held down her short, black hair. "For the first time in my life, I started to be fully present in the day I was living. I was alive. My goals were no longer long-range plans, they were daily goals, much more meaningful to me because at the end of each day, I could evaluate what I had done."

A flock of sandpipers wheeled in front of us.

"I believe that when we are fully present, we not only live well, we live well for others."

Mimi questioned her, "Why is it then, Diane, that we are so willing to give up our own authority?"

"It's easier," I interjected. "We don't have to think. The

responsibility belongs to someone else. Why are we so afraid of being selfish? And why do we distract and excuse ourselves from our own creativity?"

"Same reason," Mother replied. "It's easier. We haven't figured out that time for ourselves is ultimately time for our families. You can't be constantly giving without depleting the source. Somehow, somewhere, we must replenish ourselves."

"But that's antithetical to the culture we belong to," Mimi said. "We are taught to sacrifice, support, and endure. There are other virtues I am more interested in cultivating," she said, smiling.

"I have a joke." I said. "How does a man honor a woman?"

"I don't know—" Mother answered.

"He puts her on a pedestal and then asks her to get down on it."

Mimi laughed. Mother tried not to.

"That's terrible, Terry."

"Oh, Mother, loosen up. There's nobody spying on us— unless these rocks are bugged." I picked one up and looked underneath.

"We haven't touched our astrology charts," Mimi said, pulling out hers.

Mother and I found ours. We read each other's. We had already listened to the individual taped sessions.

"I liked the part about Terry being neat and meticulous," teased Mother. "I remember standing in the middle of your bedroom when you were about thirteen years old. Everything in your closet was on the floor, art and school papers were piled high on your desk. I remember thinking, I have two choices here—I can harp on her every day of her life, making certain her room is straight—or I can close the door and preserve our relationship."

"Thank you for choosing the latter," I said. "Brooke may feel otherwise."

"The thing that struck me about your chart, Diane," said Mimi, "was the tension in your life between your need for privacy and the obligation you feel toward your family."

"And I think I have paid a price physically," Mother said. She looked out over the lake, then back to me, "Did anything surprise you about your chart, Terry?"

"I think the part that helped me the most was recognizing that I operate with three minds. Remember when she said I can look at a teacup and say, 'Isn't this lovely, notice the pink roses on the white bone china,' or 'Isn't this fascinating, consider the cup in human history,' or 'Look at this teacup, the coffee stains and chip on its rim'—What about you, Mimi?" I asked.

"At seventy-nine, what did I learn? It was more an affirmation of what I already know. I am aware of my intense curiosity, my compulsion to understand the world around me. I value intelligence. I listened hard to those traits I have to watch. I realize I am a very frank, strong personality as a Leo, but I hope I can evolve to be a Leo with wisdom—

"I believe we must do things in our lives for the right reasons, because we enjoy doing them, with no expectation of getting something back in return. Otherwise, we are constantly being disappointed." She moved her turquoise bracelet back and forth on her wrist. "So I had two sons, John and Richard, because I wanted to, not because I thought they would rescue me in old age. I got out of all social organizations and clubs in my fifties so I could spend time with my grandchildren, not because they would give something back to Jack and me later on, but because that was what I wanted to do—and I have loved doing it. Believe me, these have been selfish decisions."

Silence followed.

Mimi looked at me. "And you, Terry?"

"I believe in facing life directly, to not be afraid of risking oneself for fear of losing too much." I paused. Here was my mother standing outside the shadow of cancer and my grandmother standing inside the threshold of old age. These were the women who had seen me through birth. These were the women I would see through death.

The three of us stared out at the lake, the color of Chinese porcelain, and were hypnotized by the waves.

"How do you find refuge in change?" I asked quietly.

Mimi put her broad hand on mine. "I don't know . . ." she whispered. "You just go with it."

A killdeer landed a few feet from where we were sitting. *"Kill-deer! Kill-deer! Kill-deer!"*

"What bird is that?" Mother asked.

"A killdeer," Mimi answered, picking up her binoculars.

I stood up to get a better look. All at once, it began to feign a broken wing, dragging it around the sand in a circle.

"Is it hurt?" Mother asked.

"No," I said. "We must be close to its nest. She's trying to distract us. It's a protective device."

"We're not so different," Mimi said, her silver hair shining in the sun. "Shall we go?"

As we got up to leave, Mother turned to me, "I'm so glad you wore your red shoes . . ."

WHISTLING SWAN

lake level: 4208.35'

The snow continues to fall. Red apples cling to bare branches.

I just returned from Tamra Crocker Pulfer's funeral. It was a reunion of childhood friends and family. Our neighborhood sat on wooden benches row after row in the chapel. I sat next to Mother and wondered how much time we had left together.

Walking the wrackline of Great Salt Lake after a storm is quite different from walking along the seashore after high tide. There are no shells, no popping kelp or crabs. What remains is a bleached narrative of feathers, bones, occasional birds encrusted in salt and deep piles of brine among the scattered driftwood. There is little human debris among the remote beaches of Great Salt Lake, except for the shotgun shells that wash up after the duck-hunting season.

Yesterday, I walked along the north shore of Stansbury Island. Great Salt Lake mirrored the plumage of immature gulls as they skimmed its surface. It was cold and windy. Small waves hissed each time they broke on shore. Up ahead, I noticed a large, white mound a few feet from where the lake was breaking.

It was a dead swan. Its body lay contorted on the beach like an abandoned lover. I looked at the bird for a long time. There was no blood on its feathers, no sight of gunshot. Most likely, a late migrant from the north slapped silly by a ravenous Great Salt Lake. The swan may have drowned.

I knelt beside the bird, took off my deerskin gloves, and began smoothing feathers. Its body was still limp—the swan had not been dead long. I lifted both wings out from under its belly and spread them on the sand. Untangling the long neck which was wrapped around itself was more difficult, but finally I was able to straighten it, resting the swan's chin flat against the shore.

The small dark eyes had sunk behind the yellow lores. It was a whistling swan. I looked for two black stones, found them, and placed them over the eyes like coins. They held. And, using my own saliva as my mother and grandmother had done to wash my face, I washed the swan's black bill and feet until they shone like patent leather.

I have no idea of the amount of time that passed in the preparation of the swan. What I remember most is lying next to its body and imagining the great white bird in flight.

I imagined the great heart that propelled the bird forward day after day, night after night. Imagined the deep breaths taken as it lifted from the arctic tundra, the camaraderie within the flock. I imagined the stars seen and recognized on clear autumn nights as they navigated south. Imagined their silhouettes passing in front of the full face of the harvest moon. And I imagined the shimmering Great Salt Lake calling the swans down like a mother, the suddenness of the storm, the anguish of its separation.

And I tried to listen to the stillness of its body.

At dusk, I left the swan like a crucifix on the sand. I did not look back.

GREAT HORNED OWL

ƒƒƒƒƒƒƒƒ

lake level: 4208.45′

"It was a perfect archetype," Mimi said of Thanksgiving in Milburn, Utah. "A log cabin in the woods with turkey on the table and four generations gathered together to pray. It couldn't be more American."

She was right. We had flocked to my aunt and uncle's place in a small, rural community. Rich and Ruth invited the entire Tempest tribe down for Thanksgiving. Twenty-six relatives arrived throughout the day.

While Mimi, Mother, and Ruth were in the kitchen preparing the feast, we children were allowed to be children again.

"Your time will come . . ." Mimi warned.

We bolted outside, seven boys and two girls, more like brothers and sisters than cousins. My cousin Lynne and I walked along the creek as our brothers went looking for deer.

"How's Diane?" she asked.

"Good," I replied. "I think it's been an adjustment for her to realize the doctors have done all they can do. The chemotherapy and radiation are over. But you can't live by your prognosis. Mom has this uncanny ability to get on with her life. I honestly think she's fine." I reached down and picked up a feather.

"Great horned owl," I said, handing it to Lynne. "Maybe tonight we can go owling. It's a full moon, you know."

We returned and joined our fathers and grandfather on the porch.

"Find anything?" Rich asked.

Lynne showed him the feather.

"Great horned," he said. He pointed to the one tucked in the band of his cowboy hat.

Lynne and I smiled. Jack took it and ran it through his fingers. "Beautiful . . ." he said, passing it on to Dad. They continued discussing state politics, Dad using the feather to accentuate his points.

"They're letting in too many out-of-state contractors," he said passionately. "There's not enough work to go around."

"And the bidding has turned into a free-for-all," added Rich.

Inside, Mimi finished making the gravy—the same recipe her grandmother had used—and announced dinner was ready. Ruth opened the back door and rang the triangle. We each found our place around the huge pine table. My uncle prayed in his deepest voice, giving thanks for all that brought us together.

"Amen," we said in unison. The platters of food were passed.

After dinner, my cousin Bob built a fire. The men stretched out on the floor and slept. Other relatives were scattered throughout the cabin.

Mother and I were washing dishes. Mimi and Ruth checked the turkey for any last filaments of meat while Lynne divided up leftovers.

"Here you go, Diane," Ruth said, handing Mother the wishbone.

Mother took the wishbone and wiped it with her towel.

"Should we let it dry or do it now?" she asked.

"Let's do it now," Lynne said.

Mother handed me the wishbone, knowing my end would break.

"Pull," she said with a mischievous smile.

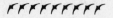

ROADRUNNER

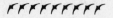

lake level: 4210.90'

I asked Mother if she would accompany me to the West Desert to check out a particular site where I was to lead a field trip for the museum. I have traded my position as curator of education for naturalist-in-residence, which means more time in the field, more time to write, and more time with Mother.

We drove west on Interstate 80 toward Nevada making fishtails on the flooded highway in Mother's Saab. Phalaropes were spinning where the median strip once was. With the sunroof open, I watched gulls. A large green sign on its way to being underwater read, GREAT SALT LAKE TEN MILES.

"I've never seen anything like this," said Mother. "What are they going to do with all this water?"

"Pump it away," I answered.

About seventy miles later, we saw where the dikes were

to be built on the salt flats. The whole country looked like a mirage against the purple backdrop of the Silver Island Range.

Only this time, it *was* the lake.

We were approaching a nine-story concrete structure, the newly erected, "Tree of Utah." Its brightly colored spheres (leaves?) resembled enormous tennis balls, thirteen feet in diameter, poised on top of an eighty-three foot lightning rod. We pulled off the freeway, got out of the car, and walked to its base.

I jumped onto the platform and read the plaque out loud: " 'Metaphor,' by Karl Momen."

We both looked at the steel tree and then at each other. This was the work of a European architect who saw the West Desert as "a large white canvas with nothing on it." This was his attempt "to put something out there to break the monotony."

With the light of morning, it cast a shadow across the salt flats like a mushroom cloud.

"Another roadside attraction in the West . . . " Mother said.

Another car stopped. We returned to ours and drove on. In the rearview mirror, the man-made tree rose from the salt flats like a small phallus dwarfed by the open space that surrounded it.

We checked into the Stateline Casino for the night. Wendover, Nevada, is to Salt Lake City what Las Vegas is to Los Angeles. Mother and I were given complimentary tickets redeemable for ten dollars worth of nickels. Mother agreed a night in front of a slot machine would be more entertaining than a movie. After settling into our room, we descended upon the casino.

We let our eyes adjust to the neon-induced darkness, the

black walls and gilded ceilings, the chaos of blips and bloops from the adjacent video arcade, and the constant ringing of bells, falling of coins, and ebullient cries of winners.

We sat at two adjacent red stools and began inserting nickels and pulling down levers. Almost instantly, Mother began winning—cherries, bells, single bars, and doubles. I inched my stool closer to the machine. Things started picking up. I didn't take my eyes off the flashing cherries. Fast and furious, we pulled the levers—simultaneously. Mother winning. Me winning. Nickels were hitting our silver trays like heavy rain. By now, my left foot was up on the counter between our two machines for leverage. Five nickels in, pull the arm down; spin, spin, spin; bar, bar, bar; nickels rain down.

A small crowd gathered.

"These women are hot!" someone yelled.

Three sevens. That's what we needed.

Five nickels in, pull the lever down, cherries roll back, forward and stop. I was communing with sevens. I could see them in my mind. *Concentrate,* I kept telling myself as I whispered to the machine, "Let go . . . let go . . ." All evening, I had been putting in five nickels for the big one-hundred-dollar pot. My eyes were glazed and my arm was loose. Five nickels, pull the lever; five nickels pull the lever; five nickels, pull the lever; one nickel, pull the lever. . .

7–7–7. Mother looked. I looked. The pit manager slapped his thigh and groaned. Two hundred nickels began dropping into the tray. Ten bucks. It could have been one hundred and the release of two thousand nickels. But on that particular whirl, I played it safe.

The pit manager offered his condolences. Mother and I laughed until we cried. Her mascara was running down her cheeks.

"There's got to be a lesson here," I said, my foot still resting on the side of the machine.

Mother pulled out her handkerchief, still laughing, and began wiping her eyes. "Oh, Terry please, just this one time, let it be bad luck!"

I received a letter from Mimi today. They are spending the winter in St. George, Utah. It reads:

Dearest Terry,

Jack has checked the mailbox every day for a week. As he was asleep this afternoon, I decided to do it myself, and there it was—clean, large, and white—your letter.

It is wonderful to hear from you. I'm so glad your time is your own now, even though there will be adjustments in your change of job.

I awakened this morning at 4:00 a.m. to see Halley's Comet. I tried to put on my slippers, robe, and jacket quietly, when suddenly I heard this voice ask, "And what may I ask are you up to?"

Jack decided to get up, too. We couldn't see the southern horizon from the porch so we decided to search for it. We were out the door by 5:15 a.m. The problem was where to go.

We tried the road to Bloomington Hills until we hit Black Road. It was a perfect view, but by this time, it was 6:00 a.m.—too late.

But what a morning. To watch the light slowly appear in the east—the colors changing moment to moment; the peach and pink of the sunrise, the deep purples, blues, and grays—I wasn't going to see Halley's Comet, but the beauty of the sky and earth were worth the effort.

I feel I need to make every effort to see "Halley." The writer Loren Eiseley made it come alive for me through his description. He had seen it as a child and hoped to see it again as a man. He died a few years ago. I feel I have to see it for him. Thank goodness, I saw the little there was in November. I have until March 22, after that the moon will be too bright.

It is in the eastern/southeastern sky, a little south of Capricornus. It's heading for the teapot. Find Aquarius, and then look directly east past Sagittarius—specifically the two stars that make up his tail. I hope you can find it. Look for both of us. And I'll do the same. In April, the comet will be very low on the horizon and difficult to see in the Mountain West.

I talked to Diane on the phone yesterday. She sounds good, busy as usual.

Terry, I think of you many times each day. Are you dreaming, dear? Send me some. It is helpful to write them down. We can discuss them over the phone if you wish.

Jack and I are feeling great and enjoying each other. After fifty-five years we understand each other so well. A fight is great now and then. It peps things up.

I'm looking forward to the Bird Refuge when we get home.

All our love,
Mimi

I saw it! Faintly above the southeastern horizon, just before dawn. Halley's Comet. A dusting of celestial particles. With my binoculars I thought I could even see its tail. It hung in the sky like a tear.

As the morning light leached into darkness, the comet vanished.

"One more time . . ." I kept whispering under my breath. "Let me see it one more time."

4210' and rising. The governor's office is once again considering pumping Great Salt Lake into the West Desert. The hopes that the breached Southern Pacific Causeway would reduce the lake and buy time until the weather subsided have been dashed.

The Utah legislature appropriated funds to conduct a required environmental impact study and develop final designs for the West Desert Pumping Project. The cost estimate revealed that the higher water level, among other factors, had increased the cost to nearly $90 million.

The project involves pumping water into a canal at the Hogup Mountain Ridge and introducing it into the salt desert, where it would spread out over a five-hundred-square-mile evaporation pond on the western side of the Newfoundland Mountains. The water in the West Desert pond would be contained by two dikes: the Bonneville Dike, approximately twenty-five miles long, which would run from Floating Island south to Interstate 80 and then along I-80 for another twelve miles; and Dike Number Two, which would extend from the southern end of the Newfoundland Mountains and run seven miles in a southeasterly direction. This dike would contain an overflow weir, which would allow the heavy, concentrated brine to flow back into the north arm of Great Salt Lake, allowing the elevation of the western pond to be varied as a means of maximizing evaporation.

The heavy brine would be allowed to flow back into the lake for two reasons. First, the evaporation rate decreases rapidly with increased salinity concentrations (the main function of the project is to evaporate water); second, the salts settling to the bottom of the evaporation pond would decrease its storage capacity and eventually decrease the viability of the project.

This month, the governor's office requested a review of the project, to determine ways to reduce the overall cost.

The new analysis reveals that a major reduction in the cost of the project could be realized by taking water from the north arm instead of constructing the diversion structure and twelve-mile canal to take water from the south arm.

This would be feasible because the salinity of the north arm has decreased from 22 percent in 1984, prior to the breach in the causeway, to 15 percent.

An additional reduction in cost has been found by assuming that the Bonneville Dike can be built at a lower elevation—and risking that the dike, under certain circumstances, would be overtopped.

These design changes reduce the overall price tag of the project from $90 million to $60 million. It is now called the "bare bones" of the West Desert Pumping Project.

"I thought the marsh would be here forever," I said to Mimi standing on the edge of the flooded Bird Refuge. Her eyes scanned Great Salt Lake.

"Things change," she said.

Afterwards, we ate lunch at the Idle Isle. Country fare in the form of mashed potatoes and gravy, pot roast, corn, and two soft dinner rolls that pull apart. It is good comfort food where nothing is complicated except the decision after the meal as to which chocolates to take home.

Mimi talked about Mother, how at fifty, women wonder what they have done with their lives. What do they believe? What is of value? What should they do with the new freedom that is theirs now that their children are, for the most part, grown?

"It's a wonderful time in a woman's life to really explore the possibilities. Your mother has changed a great deal over the years." Mimi said. "And I think her cancer had a lot to do with it. During the early 1970s when many women were rethinking their roles within the home and confronting their own independence, I saw Diane focusing on her health, living, surviving, so she could raise you children. Along the way, she became much more philosophical. I admire how she protects her energy and understands her limitations."

"What was it like when your mother passed away?" I asked Mimi.

"I was twenty-eight years old. I had just given birth to John when I found out Mother had died from a stomach ulcer. A sudden infection. She had just made plans to come from Washington, D.C. to see him."

She paused.

"I'll never forget the telegram my sister Marion sent. I couldn't believe it. It was so final. Suddenly, the world seemed very dark. I couldn't imagine how I was going to live without her and I grieved deeply that she was never able to see her first grandchild. But I will tell you, Terry, you do get along. It isn't easy. The void is always with you. But you will get by without your mother just fine and I promise you, you will become stronger and stronger each day."

Mother. She is preoccupied. Yesterday, on the telephone, she said she didn't think she could make the family backpacking trip in the Tetons scheduled for summer.

"I think I may have pulled some muscles in my stomach," she said.

I want to believe her.

It rains and rains. Great Salt Lake continues to rise.

Eudora Welty, when asked what causes she would support, replied, "Peace, education, conservation, and quiet."

Mother, Mimi and Jack, and I are seeking quiet in St. George, Utah.

Early this morning, we decided against our planned hike to Beaver Dam Wash in the Mojave Desert. At dawn, another nuclear bomb was being detonated underground at the Nevada Test Site.

Mimi and I were in the living room reading, Jack was outside, when Mother exclaimed from the kitchen, "They're here!"

We ran out on the balcony. It was a slow-moving river, hundreds of people walking on behalf of nuclear disarmament. The Great Peace March. We left the house to greet them.

Up the hill toward Green Valley, they walked by us—a procession of children, parents, and grandparents.

"I could join them," Mother said under her breath as we clapped for them.

A song rose up from the activists:

> *We are a gentle, loving people*
> *and we are walking, walking for our lives—*

We walked with them. It was the first time I had ever heard Mother and Mimi sing outside of church.

From the corner of my eye, I saw a roadrunner poised on the desert. I have never considered them to be a patriotic bird, but with its patch of red, white, and blue skin painted like a flag on the side of its head, I looked at him differently.

MAGPIES

lake level: 4211.30'

The Mormon Church declared Sunday, May 5, 1986, a day of prayer on behalf of the weather; that the rains might be stopped. The "Citizens for the Return of Lake Bonneville" also declared it a day of prayer; that the rains might continue. Each organization viewed the other as a cult.

Monday, it rained.

Flocks of magpies have descended on our yard. I cannot sleep for all their raucous behavior. Perched on weathered fences, their green-black tails, long as rulers, wave up and down, reprimanding me for all I have not done.

I have done nothing for weeks. I have no work. I don't want to see anyone much less talk. All I want to do is sleep.

Monday, I hit rock-bottom, different from bedrock which is solid, expansive, full of light and originality.

Rock-bottom is the bottom of the rock, the underbelly that rarely gets turned over; but when it does, I am the spider that scurries from daylight to find another place to hide.

Today, I feel stronger, learning to live within the natural cycles of a day and to not expect so much from myself. As women, we hold the moon in our bellies. It is too much to ask to operate on full-moon energy three hundred and sixty-five days a year. I am in a crescent phase. And the energy we expend emotionally belongs to the hidden side of the moon.

Mother called from St. George. Yesterday, she hiked alone in Zion National Park. Finally, she has her solitude. Her voice was radiant. "Until you go through this process of facing death, or the probability of it—no one can ever know there is something that takes its place. It goes beyond hope."

Mother's whole being is accelerated. I see her insatiable curiosity intensify. Her desire to absorb everything that is fresh and natural and alive is magnified. She is the bird touching both heaven and earth, flying with newfound knowledge of what it means to live. She is reading Zen, Krishnamurti, and Jung, asking herself questions she has never had the courage to explore. Suddenly, the shackles which have bound her are beginning to snap, as personal revelation replaces orthodoxy.

"When I get home, we'll have a chaparral tea party," Mother said. "It's supposed to strengthen your immune system. I'm drinking some now. It looks like a drug stash."

Her inner retreat of the past few months has momentarily been replaced by openness.

"It's all inside," she said. "I just needed to get away, to be reminded by the desert of who I am and who I am not. The exposed geologic layers in the redrock mirror the depths within myself."

She paused over the phone.

"Remember when I asked you what you believed in?"

I nodded and took her bait. "Yes," I said. "So what do you believe, Mother?"

"I believe in me."

Last night, I spoke at one of the Circle Meetings of the Baptist Church. Afterward, a Kenyan friend, Wangari Waigwa-Stone, and I spoke about darkness and stars.

"I was raised under an African sky," she said. "Darkness was never something I was afraid of. The clarity, definition, and profusion of stars became maps as to how one navigates at night. I always knew where I was simply by looking up." She paused. "My sons do not have these guides. They have no relationship to darkness, nothing in their imagination tells them there are pathways in the night they can move through."

"I have a Norwegian friend who says, 'City lights are a conspiracy against higher thought,' " I added.

"Indeed," Wangari said, smiling, her rich, deep voice resonating. "I am Kikuyu. My people believe if you are close to the Earth, you are close to people."

"How so?" I asked.

"What an African woman nurtures in the soil will eventually feed her family. Likewise, what she nurtures in her relations will ultimately nurture her community. It is a matter of living the circle.

"Because we have forgotten our kinship with the land," she continued, "our kinship with each other has become pale. We shy away from accountability and involvement. We choose to be occupied, which is quite different from being engaged. In America, time is money. In Kenya, time is relationship. We look at investments differently."

"It all comes down to dollars and cents," Dad said over the phone this morning.

"I've got a tip from Mountain Fuel. It looks like the governor is going ahead with the West Desert Pumping Project. Thirty-seven miles of six-inch pipe will have to be laid for the natural-gas line to fuel the pumps. The line will run from a site near AMAX's plant to the pumping station near Hogup Ridge. If Mountain Fuel is awarded the $2.7 million contract to build the transmission line to supply power for the pumps, they'll open it for bidding within the next couple of months. I want to take a look at the country so it's in my mind before we actually start figuring footage. Do you want to drive out with me?"

I was delighted to get out.

No drive to the West Desert is simple, especially one to the west shore of Great Salt Lake. We took I-80, turned north toward Lakeside, and then bumped along dirt roads until Dad decided it was time to stretch out and walk.

"You've got to get a feel for the land before you can lay the pipe," he said. "Nothing is as it appears. What do you see?"

We stood on a ridge of the Hogup Mountains.

"I see miles and miles of salt flats and sage, greasewood, and shadescale."

"How does the digging look to you?"

"It looks fairly easy, not that much rock."

"That's where you'd get into trouble."

We hiked off the ridge toward the salt flats. Dad's pace was brisk. What appeared to be an easy walk took several hours. Dad began digging a test hole. The hole filled with water.

"The water table, of course." I mused.

"Exactly," he said. "Because of the lake level, these flats are saturated. You have to build that into your costs."

He dug a few more. Same results.

"I'd love to get this job," he said, his eyes squinting from the sun. "It would be exciting to be part of this project, even though I think the whole concept is ridiculous. We'll pump the lake into places it had no intention of going . . . the lake will recede and then what will be left?"

"What would happen," I asked, "if the governor said, 'I've decided to do nothing. Great Salt Lake is cyclic. This is a natural phenomenon. Our roads are built on a flood plain. We will move them.' " I looked at my father.

"He'd be impeached," Dad said, laughing. "The lakeshore industry is hurting financially. The pumping project is a way to bail out the salt and mineral companies, Southern Pacific Railroad, and a political career as well."

"Or ruin one . . ." I said.

"Politicians don't understand that the land, the water, the air, all have minds of their own. I understand it because I work with the elements every day. Our livelihood depends on it. If it rains, we quit. If it's a hundred degrees outside, our men suffer. And when the ground freezes, we can't lay pipe. If we don't make adjustments with the environment, our company goes broke." He looked out over the huge body of water glistening with salt crystals. "Sure, this lake has a mind, but it cares nothing for ours."

A special session of the Utah legislature was called to authorize $60 million for the construction and operation of the West Desert Pumping Project. The okay was given, the funds released, with the first pump slated to begin its job of bailing Great Salt Lake out to the desert in February 1987.

A deep sadness washes over me for all that has been lost. The water level of Great Salt Lake is so high now that it recalls the memory and reality of Lake Bonneville. The Wasatch Mountains capped with snow seem to rise from a sparkling blue sea.

I am not adjusting. I keep dreaming the Refuge back to what I have known: rich, green bulrushes that border the wetlands, herons hidden behind cattails, concentric circles of ducks on ponds. I blow on these images like the last burning embers on a winter's night.

There is no one to blame, nothing to fight. No developer with a dream of condominiums. No toxic waste dump that would threaten the birds. Not even a single dam on the Bear River to oppose. Only a simple natural phenomenon: the rise of Great Salt Lake.

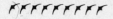

LONG-BILLED
CURLEWS

lake level: 4211.65'

It is snowing at Bear River in May. I can only drive out three miles west of Brigham City. The lake stops me. Before the flood, it was a fifteen mile trip. The waves of Great Salt Lake are lapping just below where my car door opens. Gray sky. Gray water. I have the sense that I am suspended in the middle of the lake with pelicans, coots, and grebes. I keep driving with the illusion that my old Peugeot station wagon is really a boat. When the lake starts seeping into the floor-boards, I come to my senses. I stop the car, carefully open the door and climb on to the roof.

Today's storm has brought in the birds. Everywhere I look, wind and wings. Swarms of swallows dip down at the crest of each wave to feed. Ibises, avocets, and stilts forage in the submerged grasses. Geese fly above them, and it is unclear whether snowflakes fall or feathers. It is one of those curious days when time and season are out of focus, when what you know is hidden behind the weather.

I return the next day to find clear skies and fewer birds. Instead, it is midge heaven with dead carp heaved on the road by the waves of yesterday's storm. The smell is foul, but it doesn't seem to bother the fishermen. I have joined them with my low-rider lawn chair. We are evenly spaced like herons along the banks of the Bear River.

This is a heavily used area a few miles west of Brigham City, known to locals as "First River." It smells of stale fish eggs and trash. Broken slabs of concrete litter the ground. But it's the only place left near the Refuge to watch birds.

Unless you have a raft.

I watch two western grebes through my binoculars. Their eyes are rubies against white feathers. The male's black head-feathers are flared and flattened on top, so they resemble Grace Jones. The female is impressed as she swims alongside. All at once, they arch their backs, extend their necks, and dash across the flat water with great speed and grace. They sink back down. They rise up again, running across the water. They sink back down.

This is the western grebes' "water rush," their courtship dance that ensures the species. I brought along Julian Huxley's *The Courtship Habits of the Great Crested Grebe* to read by the river, just in case there were no birds.

After the grebes retreat into the bulrushes, I flip through the small book, stopping at Huxley's description of the "weed-trick ceremony."

> Taken all in all, the courtship is chiefly mutual and self-exhausting, the excitatory, sexual form of courtship such as weed offering or pure display serve not as exci-

tants to coition, as in most birds, but as excitants to some further act of courtship.

Although Huxley writes about European cousins to the western grebes, family characteristics are hard to shake. What great-crested grebes do, western grebes do also.

The two grebes I have been watching, white-throated and black-backed, begin circling one another and bobbing their heads. Between head-shakes, the male rolls his neck on to his back and seductively preens feathers.

Huxley describes this behavior to a tee: "The simplest form of courtship action is the bout of shaking . . ." Huxley elaborates:

> Shaking may take place either before or after courtship actions . . . it varies a certain amount in intensity and in length and also in the amount of habit-preening that takes place . . . each bird excites the other. One gently shakes its head under the force of rising emotional tension; the other bird had not quite got to that stage, but the sight of its mate shaking acts as a stimulus, and it too pricks up its head a little and gives a shake. This reacts on the first bird, and so the excitement is mutually increased and the process fulfills itself.

I am a voyeur. The fisherman to my left asks me if I have been here before. Without thinking, I turn to the man and shake my head in a rather grebelike way, then immediately blush, hoping he has not been watching the amorous birds and mistaken my behavior as flirtatious.

I decide to walk along the river's edge. I stir up clouds of midges. They rise in thick black columns that sound like the string section of an orchestra holding one note as the bow moves frantically back and forth across the bridge. I take a few steps, and the winged column narrows as they raise their pitch another octave.

Through my binoculars, in a continued scan, I spot three wrecked cars, one nose down in the cattails, a Pontiac with a great blue heron standing on its tail lights. There is a spray of gunshot. The heron flies. Three ibises spring up, then float back down into the grasses. I turn. Suddenly, I feel as vulnerable as the long-legged birds.

On my way home, I stop at a favorite pond to watch a pair of cinnamon teals. Barn swallows fly in and out from under the bridge. Dozens of nests are plastered with mud against the concrete beam. A barn swallow is busy lining its cuplike nest with white down feathers. It flies, returning seconds later, with another piece of down in its beak. I wonder where the cache is—most likely a goose nest.

The cliff swallows' nests are different from the barn swallows', although both are built beneath the bridge. Their nests are enclosed, with a small hole left open as an entrance. One pair, their nest barely a shelf, takes turns bringing back dabs of mud. Ten dabs of mud in five minutes. Within an hour, I watch them pack 120 beak-loads of mud onto their new residence. The swallows tirelessly fly to the mudflats on the edge of the pond, load up their bills, return to the construction site, vibrate their heads as they pour the mud onto the nest. Then they vigorously pat it and shape it around their nest. They alternate turns as the male flies from the nest to the mudflat, loads, while the female pats. He returns, she flies out. Over and over again, the same painstaking work, as their tiny feathered bodies quiver with purpose. The shelf slowly, steadily, becomes a closed dwelling.

The spinning of phalaropes. The courtship of grebes. The growth of a swallow's nest. Each—a natural history unfolding.

North of Promontory Point, where the golden spike commemorated the completion of the transcontinental railroad on May 10, 1869, there is a remote vale called Curlew Valley. It is the breeding ground of the long-billed curlew.

In recent years, the long-billed curlew, the largest North American shorebird, has been declining in number in the Great Basin, as it loses much of its breeding habitat to the plow and other land developments. In the midwest, it has been extirpated as a breeding species altogether.

The eskimo curlew is close to extinction. At the turn of the century, in its northward migrations a single flock covered forty to fifty acres in the grasslands of Nebraska. They were known as "prairie pigeons" or "dough birds." As wagonloads were shot and sold, they took the place of the passenger pigeon on the marketplace. Hunters followed the curlews' migration from state to state, literally making a killing. Those who remember the eskimo curlew's call say it sounded like "the wind whistling through a ship's rigging."

If grasslands continue to shrink, the long-billed curlew could follow the same path as its relative. Its plaintive cry resounds like a warning.

Long-billed curlew, *Numenius americanus,* takes its genus from the Greek *neos,* meaning "new" and *mene,* "moon." The shape of its long bill was thought to resemble the curvature of the sliver moon.

If new moon is defined as no moon or dark moon, the curlew could be associated with destructive powers, for it was long believed that ghosts, goblins, and witches were at the peak of their power in the dark of the moon.

In folklore, this relationship between curlews and black magic stands. A prayer of the Scottish Highlands asks "to be saved from witches, warlocks, and aw lang-nebbed things." In Scotland, the word *whaup* is the name of both the curlew and a goblin with a long beak who moves about under the eaves of attics at night.

In *The Folklore of Birds,* Edward Armstrong writes, "Flocks of curlews, passing over at night and uttering their plaintive, musical calls have also been regarded as the Seven Whistlers, and in the north of England their voices were said to presage someone's death."

He goes on to say, "The curlew's low-pitched fluting is sufficiently near the range of human voice to arouse in the heart the sense of weirdness which we are apt to feel on hearing sounds which have some simulation to but do not really belong to the world of men."

Curlews have been seen as winged souls with foreboding messages. Curiosities of natural history have been defined by curlews. An old-timer of the moors once told a friend of mine there was always an accident after hearing "them long-billed curlews." He spoke of a flock passing overhead and, a few minutes later, their boat overturned. Seven men drowned.

But the flipside of darkness is light. The new moon is also the resurrected moon, soon to be crescent, quarter, then full. It is the time in many cultures to sow seeds. During the waxing moon all those things that needed to grow are attended to.

In the dark of the moon there is growth. Plants do not flourish in the noonday sun, but rather in the privacy of the new moon.

Maybe it is not the darkness we fear most, but the silences contained within the darkness. Maybe it is not the absence of the moon that frightens us, but the absence of what we expect to be there. A wedge of long-billed curlews flying in the night punctuates the silences and their unexpected calls remind us the only thing we can expect is change.

I found the long-billed curlews at Curlew Valley. A dozen hovered over me like banshees,

"Cur-lee! Cur-lee! Cur-lee!"

I was in their territory and they did not like it. Because of their camouflage, those in the grasses were difficult to see. Movement was my only clue. I counted seven adults. Most were pecking and probing the overgrazed landscape, plucking out multitudes of grasshoppers in between the stubble. Others were contesting the boundaries of competing curlews as they chased each other with heads low in a running crouch. Two curlews faced each other, with necks extended, their long bills pointing toward the sky. They looked ready to fence. Tense gestures, until one bird backed down and flew. The triumphant curlew stepped forward and fluttered its strong, pointed wings above its head. Cinnamon underfeathers flashed like the bright slip of a Spanish dancer.

Female curlews, slightly larger than the males, were prostrate, their necks stretched outward from their bodies. I suspected they were on nests and did not disturb them.

Burr buttercups grew between the grasses like snares, and in prairie dogs' abandoned holes black widows, the size of succulent grapes, reigned.

The hostility of this landscape teaches me how to be quiet and unobtrusive, how to find grace among spiders with a poisonous bite. I sat on a lone boulder in the midst of the curlews. By now, they had grown accustomed to me. This too, I found encouraging—that in the face of stressful intrusions, we can eventually settle in. One begins to almost trust the intruder as a presence that demands greater intent toward life.

On a day like today when the air is dry and smells of salt, I have found my open space, my solitude, and sky. And I have found the birds who require it.

There is something unnerving about my solitary travels around the northern stretches of Great Salt Lake. I am never entirely at ease because I am aware of its will. Its mood can change in minutes. The heat alone reflecting off the salt is enough to drive me mad, but it is the glare that immobilizes me. Without sunglasses, I am blinded. My eyes quickly burn on Salt Well Flats. It occurs to me that I will return home with my green irises bleached white. If I return at all.

The understanding that I could die on the salt flats is no great epiphany. I could die anywhere. It's just that in the foresaken corners of Great Salt Lake there is no illusion of being safe. You stand in the throbbing silence of the Great Basin, exposed and alone. On these occasions, I keep tight reins on my imagination. The pearl-handed pistol I carry in my car lends me no protection. Only the land's mercy and a calm mind can save my soul. And it is here I find grace.

It's strange how deserts turn us into believers. I believe in walking in a landscape of mirages, because you learn humility. I believe in living in a land of little water because life is drawn together. And I believe in the gathering of bones as a testament to spirits that have moved on.

If the desert is holy, it is because it is a forgotten place that allows us to remember the sacred. Perhaps that is why every pilgrimage to the desert is a pilgrimage to the self. There is no place to hide, and so we are found.

In the severity of a salt desert, I am brought down to my knees by its beauty. My imagination is fired. My heart opens and my skin burns in the passion of these moments. I will have no other gods before me.

Wilderness courts our souls. When I sat in church throughout my growing years, I listened to teachings about Christ in the wilderness for forty days and forty nights, reclaiming his strength, where he was able to say to Satan, "Get thee hence." When I imagined Joseph Smith kneeling in a grove of trees as he received his vision to create a new religion, I believed their sojourns into nature were sacred. Are ours any less?

There is a Mormon scripture, from the Doctrine and Covenants section 88:44–47, that I carry with me:

> The earth rolls upon her wings, and the sun giveth
>   his light by day, and the moon giveth her light
>   by night, and the stars also give their light, as
>   they roll upon their wings in their glory, in the
>   midst of the power of God.
> Unto what shall I liken these kingdoms that ye may
>   understand?
> Behold all these are kingdoms and any man who
>   hath seen any or the least of these hath seen God
>   moving in his majesty and power.

I pray to the birds.

I pray to the birds because I believe they will carry the messages of my heart upward. I pray to them because I believe in their existence, the way their songs begin and end each day—the invocations and benedictions of Earth. I pray to the birds because they remind me of what I love rather than what I fear. And at the end of my prayers, they teach me how to listen.

Hundreds of white pelicans appear—white against blue. They turn, disappear. Reappear, black against blue. They turn, disappear. Reappear, white against blue. Through my binoculars, I can see their bright orange bills, many with the characteristic knobs associated with courtship.

The grassy banks of Teal Spring are a welcome reprieve from the barren country I have come from. This is just one of the many small ponds at Locomotive Springs, ten miles from Curlew Valley. It is classified by the Utah Division of Wildlife Resources as a "first-magnitude marsh," which means a place with a stable water supply used by waterfowl for nesting, migration, and wintering. I would call it a first-magnitude marsh simply because it's green.

Brooke will come later this evening. Until then, I shall curl up in the grasses like a bedded animal and dream.

Marsh music. Red-wing blackbirds. Yellow-headed blackbirds. Song sparrows. Barn swallows snapping mosquitoes on the wing. Herons traversing the sky.

Brooke arrives and we walk.

The sign TEAL SPRING is silhouetted against a numinous sky. Its reflection in the pond looks like a black cross. We listen to the catcall of a redhead. Thousands of birds seem to be speaking behind us. We turn around and find only a fortress of greasewood.

Settling into our sleeping bag, I nestle into Brooke's body. We are safe. With our arms around each other, we watch ibis after ibis, heron after heron, teal after teal, fly over us. A few stars appear. We try counting them, until finally the sweet whimperings of shorebirds seduce us into sleep.

Sunrise. Teal Spring is transformed. The pinks and lavenders of the night before have been exchanged for the vitality of yellows and blues. Even the rushes, whose black reflection bled into the water twelve hours earlier, are golden. Instead of the stalks predominating, morning light has struck their flowering heads like a match. Small flames flicker on each tip.

To spend a night at the marsh is to wax and wane with birdsong. At sunset and for an hour or so afterward, the pitch and frenzy of birds is so high, so frantic, idle conversation is impossible. But after midnight, silence. The depth and stillness of Great Salt Lake comes over the wetlands like a mother's calming hand. Morning approaches slowly, until each voice in the marsh awakens.

Brooke and I walk miles across the northwestern wetlands and alkaline flats of the lake. Salt crystals attached to the mud look like blistered skin. The sun is searing and the black gnats are almost intolerable. Relief comes only through concentration, losing ourselves in the studied behavior of birds.

Marbled godwits forage the flats with avocets and stilts. It would be easy to confuse the godwits with curlews, except for their bicolored bills that point upward, not down. And I find their character very different from curlews—more trusting, more gentle, more calm. When a curlew is near, the air is stirred; they are anxious and aggressive. Godwits are serene. They demand little from you except the patience to observe. Curlews cause guilt. You are reminded of your intrusion, that you do not belong.

As we walked along an eroding dike, flush with the roaring lake, a blue heron flies off its nest leaving four large eggs. The nest is built of dried greasewood on an old weathered fence that fans out like an accordion. Two ravens hover with eyes on the eggs. We leave quickly, so the heron can return.

Walking back toward Teal Spring, we discover a dead curlew. Its body lies fixed, encrusted with salt. We kneel down and run our fingers down its long, curved bill. Brooke ponders over the genetic information a species is born with, the sophistication of cells and the memory held inside a gene pool. It is the embryology of a curlew that informs the stubby, straight beak of a chick to take a graceful curve down.

I say a silent prayer for the curlew, remembering the bond of two days before when I sat in their valley nurtured by solitude. I ask the curlew for cinnamon-barred feathers and take them.

They do not come easily.

WESTERN TANAGER

lake level: 4211.85'

4211.85'. Great Salt Lake has surpassed its historic high of 1873. The date is June 2, 1986. It is also our anniversary. Eleven years.

Brooke and I vigorously shake a bottle of champagne, pull the cork, and let it spray into the salty waters of the south shore. With dripping hands, Brooke pours the champagne into the crystal goblets I hold.

"Don't worry about me in the coming months," he says. "I know where you need to be."

We toast to marriage and the indomitable spirit of Great Salt Lake.

I find that the time with Mother is spent in quiet reflection, oftentimes, talking from our trips across the desert.

Last weekend, we were driving home from St. George. As we were passing through Provo, Utah, the town where she was born, she turned to me.

"I just remembered the strangest thing from my childhood . . ."

"What is that?" I asked.

"I remember walking home from school one afternoon and seeing Mother and Dad standing in front of our house. I could see in their faces that something was wrong. As I walked up to the door, Dad said, 'Diane, Blackie was hit by a car.' They put their arms around me and cried. What they had just said to me did not seem real. I asked if I could see him. They told me they had buried him in the backyard while I was at school. Mother explained that she didn't want me to have to see my dog that way. In their minds, they had protected me from one of life's sorrows."

"That night, I remember sneaking out of the house in my nightgown, trying to find the place where they had buried my black lab. I found the disturbed soil, knelt on the damp grass and began digging with my bare hands to uncover him. I wanted to see his broken body. I wanted to cradle his bones and see for myself that he was dead. I wanted to cry over the death of my dog. But the hole was too deep and I never found him."

"Isn't that funny I would remember that incident after all these years?"

"Why do you think?" I asked.

"What are you saying?" Mother sounded puzzled.

"I don't know—maybe there is something in that story that you need right now, maybe that's why it surfaced."

Mother turned her head. From the corner of my eye, I saw her staring out her window.

"Maybe I have never been allowed to grieve. Maybe I have never allowed myself to grieve."

"There is no blockage as of now, Diane. We can try another type of chemotherapy called Leukeran, different from the cisplatin and Cytoxan you had two years ago. There's a chance it might shrink the tumor we've found."

"And if I do nothing?" Mother asked.

Dr. Smith looked over at me. I raised my eyebrows to indicate that I was simply a bystander.

"A blockage will occur. I don't know how soon, but you will not be able to eat. At that point, I think you will want the blockage removed—so there may be more surgery—but let's not get ahead of ourselves."

He paused. "You don't think you want to try Leukeran?"

"No," Mother said.

He paused again.

"I respect that. Let's just see how things go, then. Diane, I had hoped—"

"I know," she broke in. "I just want to be able to continue in the decision making. I'm not afraid of my own death, but I am afraid of the pain." She hesitated. "I hope I have the courage to face what's ahead."

"You do," he said. "Call me when you think I can help." Dr. Smith walked us to the door.

Mother turned to him and took his hand, "Thank you. You have been wonderful."

We left the clinic. I looked at Mother and asked how she could remain so strong.

"Tell me, Terry, what choice do I have?"

Mother has chosen not to say anything to Dad and the family until after Hank's birthday, not because she doesn't want them to know, but because she wants to protect herself.

"I don't want everyone hovering over me as though I have a day or two to live. Besides, this is terribly boring."

"I'm not sure I would use the word, boring . . ."

"Illness is boring," she said. "Take my word."

"You seem to have a different attitude, Mother. Is that true?"

"It feels good to finally be able to embrace my cancer. It's almost like a friend," she said. "For the first time, I feel like moving with it and not resisting what is ahead. Before, I always knew I had more time, that the disease was outside of myself. This time, I don't feel that way. The cancer is very much a part of me."

"Terry, I need you to help me through my death."

I laid my head on her lap and closed my eyes. I could not tell if it was my mother's fingers combing through my hair or the wind.

The Bear River Migratory Bird Refuge offices officially closed today, according to the U.S. Fish and Wildlife area supervisor in Denver.

"We have pretty well abandoned the sixty-five-thousand-acre refuge fourteen miles west of Brigham City, because it is impossible to second-guess the Great Salt Lake," said Phil Norton. He explained that the maintenance worker assigned to the Refuge is being transferred to the Fish Springs Refuge, near Dugway in Tooele County. Peter Smith, acting manager of Bear River, will be reassigned with the Denver district, and a part-time secretary will be looking for a job.

At its peak, Mr. Norton said, the Bird Refuge "employed eight full-time people and four seasonal workers." Refuge employees began preparing for high waters from the Great Salt Lake in 1983. The press release cited "most of the

fourteen-mile-long blacktop road to the Refuge as underwater," and Box Elder county commissioner chairman
James W. White said, "At today's prices, it will cost $1
million a mile to elevate and repair the road . . ."

During an inspection trip a month ago, Mr. Norton and
Mr. Smith reported, "more than $150,000 worth of damage
had been done to the government buildings as a result of the
wind blowing large chunks of ice off the lake into the
structures."

Bear River now belongs to the birds.

On July 1, 1986, I cooked my first turkey for Hank's
twentieth birthday. Brooke came home from work last
night and found it soaking in the bathtub. I had forgotten
to take it out of the freezer. I wanted Mother to know I
could carry out the family traditions, that Thanksgiving and
Christmas would be in good hands. It didn't work. The
turkey was terrible.

Even so, there was a warmth and closeness to the evening.
No one else knew about Mother. We all knew. Sometimes
it is appropriate to skate on surfaces.

Dawn to dusk. I have spent the entire day with
Mother. Lying next to her. Rubbing her back. Holding her
fevered hand close to my face. Stroking her hair. Keeping
ice on the back of her neck. She is so uncomfortable. We
are trying to work with the pain.

Her jaw tightens. She cramps. And then she breathes.

I am talking her through a visualization, asking her to
imagine what the pain looks like, what color it is, to lean
into the sensation rather than resisting it. We breathe
through the meditation together.

The light begins to deepen. It is sunset. I open the shutters, so Mother can see the clouds. I return to her bedside. She takes my hand and whispers, "Will you give me a blessing?"

In Mormon religion, formal blessings of healing are given by men through the Priesthood of God. Women have no outward authority. But within the secrecy of sisterhood we have always bestowed benisons upon our families.

Mother sits up. I lay my hands upon her head and in the privacy of women, we pray.

It's the Fourth of July, and the family decides to celebrate in the Tetons. Mother says she is sick of lying in bed and needs a change of scenery. I wonder how far she can push herself.

Brooke and I, with Mother and Dad, hike to Taggart Lake.

The Taggart-Bradley fire of last fall has opened up the country. It is a garden of wildflowers with fireweed, spirea, harebell, lupine, and heart-leaf arnica shimmering against the charred bark of lodgepole pines.

I have never been aware of the creek's path until now. It feels good to be someplace lush. The salt desert is too stark for me now because my interior is bare.

We reach the lake, only a mile and a half away, but each step for Mother is a triumph of will. She rests on her favorite boulder, a piece of granite I have known since childhood. She leans into the shade of the woods and closes her eyes.

"This feels so good," she says as the wind circles her. "It feels so good to be cool. I feel like I'm burning up inside."

A western tanager, red, yellow, and black, flies to the low branch of a lodgepole.

"Look, Mother! A tanager!" I hand her my binoculars.

"You look for me . . ." she says.

GRAY JAYS

lake level: 4211.40'

I am retreating into the Wasatch Mountains. I cannot travel west to Great Salt Lake. It is too exposed, too wicked and hot with one-hundred degree temperatures. The granite of Big Cottonwood Canyon invigorates me as I hike from Brighton to Lake Catherine. Glacier lilies blanket the meadows. Usually they are gone by now. I pick one and press it between the pages of my journal.

"For Mother—" I say to myself, rationalizing my act, when I know it is for me.

Hiking the narrow trail up the steep slope massages my lungs. I breathe deeply. Inhale. Exhale. Inhale. Exhale.

I climb up the last pass and break down into the cirque. My lungs and legs feel strong. I have the lake to myself. My ears begin to throb with the altitude. My eyes water in the wind. I take off my rucksack, pull out my windbreaker and lunch. I can see the rock I am going to sit on. I hike down a little further and settle in.

Peeling an orange is a good thing to do in the mountains. It slows you down. You bite into the tart rind, pull it back with your teeth and then let your fingers undress the citrus. Nothing else exists beyond or before this task. The naked fruit is in your hands waiting for sections to be separated. Halves. Quarters. And then the delicacy of breaking the orange down to its smallest smile.

I lay out these ten sections on the flat granite rock I am sitting on. The sun threatens to dry them. But I wait for the birds. Within minutes, Clark's nutcrackers and gray jays join me. I suck on oranges as the mountains begin to work on me.

This is why I always return. This is why I can always go home.

I brought the pressed glacier lily to Mother. I found her sitting in the chaise lounge on the porch with a glass of ice water in her hand. It has been almost a week since she has been able to eat.

Mother turned around. As she took the flower, she said, "Terry, what I have to do now goes beyond the family."

The Tempest clan met for a family portrait. Everyone: Mimi and Jack, Mother and Dad, Richard and Ruth, all nine grandchildren with spouses, plus two great-grandchildren. A large elm with ivy winding around its trunk stood regally in the background. It was all very formal. Nobody wanted to be there. It was my idea. I thought it would be a nice Christmas present for Mimi and Jack. The photographer framed us with his hands, then disappeared behind his black broadcloth.

"Smile!" he yelled. "You all look so somber. What's the matter, is somebody dying?"

We lost control. Laughs turned into tears into sidesplitting hysteria. Richard looked at Dad who looked at Mother who looked at Mimi who looked at Jack, and so on down the family.

The photographer stepped out from behind the camera and shook his head. "Did I say something funny?"

Mother is in surgery. Brooke brought us lunch. The men are talking politics. Dad is figuring a bid. Hank is writing. Steve and Dan are walking the halls. Again.

We wait.

I am suspended between the past and future, held by a spider's filament stretched across a river.

Five twenty-five P.M. My concentration snaps as the doctor enters.

"She's fine." he says. "We removed the blockage. It was at the very end of her small intestine, a much better situation than we anticipated. There is still a sprinkling of cancer cells, but we can work with them."

Dr. Smith looks at my father.

"Maybe a year . . ."

"You still don't understand, do you?" Mother said to me. "It doesn't matter how much time I have left. All we have is now. I wish you could all accept that and let go of your projections. Just let me live so I can die."

Her words cut through me like broken glass. This afternoon, she said, "Terry, to keep hoping for life in the midst of letting go is to rob me of the moment I am in."

We had a slide show in Mother's hospital room. Brooke projected all the different takes of the family portrait on the white wall. We needed Mother's help in deciding which image was the best of everyone. We also brought chocolate cake, ice cream, and balloons, because it was Dad's birthday.

Mother wasn't interested.

We raised her bed so she could see the pictures. Finally, she asked to be returned to a horizontal position and simply said, "They all look fine."

The party ended early. Dad, Brooke, and I stayed. The men decided to take a walk outside the hospital. Mother was asleep, her breathing labored. I pulled a chair close to the side of her bed and began quietly breathing with her, emphasizing each exhale.

Almost an hour passed.

Dad and Brooke returned. I stood up and moved the chair back against the wall.

"She looks more relaxed," Dad said.

Brooke looked at me. We kissed her and left.

Mother does not seem to be getting better. Her spirit has turned inward. She has little energy for others. Even the gardenia by her bedside that once brought her great pleasure offers little solace.

Dad and I decide what Mother needs, after fourteen days in a small, square room with little light, is fresh air. Without asking the nurses' or doctor's permission, we sneak her out of the hospital. Gathering all the bottles, bags, and tubing necessary for transport, we wheeled her outside.

It was a glorious summer day with huge cumulus clouds towering over the Wasatch. We took Mother to some gardens of pansies and marigolds. The heat seemed to draw color back in to her pale cheeks and, for the first time in weeks, her eyes brightened.

Dad sat on the grass beside her wheelchair talking in soft tones about the beauty before her, tenderly rubbing her legs. She began to cry from the soles of her feet.

We sat in the sunshine for an hour or more, until she said she was ready to go back inside.

"Thank you."

Dad was wheeling Mother back toward the hospital when a large black dog appeared. We stopped. Mother put out her hand. The labrador licked her palm and then laid his head in her lap. She lifted her other hand from the armrest and gently stroked his head.

At last, my mother grieved.

Mother is home from the hospital. A neighbor who had seen the lights on in the bedroom at midnight brought over some hot, homemade custard. Dad took the glass bowl out to the balcony to cool and brought it back inside when it was comfortably warm. He fed it to Mother. She ate. We stood at the foot of their bed and watched. She had not been able to eat for almost four weeks, until now.

"Delicious . . ." Mother said cooing. "It's absolutely delicious."

These summer days have been relentless with emotional heat. I am exhausted and depleted. This afternoon when I was taking Mother her pain medication, the doorbell rang, and without thinking, I took the pill myself. Standing on the front porch were women from the Relief Society with dinner for the family. It wasn't until Mother asked moments later for the Percodan that I realized what I had done.

She is exhausted from the weeks of sustained pain, and tonight I realized it could be months. Every day is a crisis because our expectations make it so.

"When will I ever feel good again?" Mother asked.

That is the question we are all living.

Steve has been massaging her forehead between pain contractions that come in intervals as predictable as labor. Dan gives her a sponge bath with ice water on the hour to break the fever. I watch our family fight the undertow of grief.

When I left to kiss Mother good-bye for the day, I noticed she was wearing two strands of heishe and pipestone around her neck, not her customary pearls.

"Hank," she said with a grin. "He gave me his medicine beads when I got home yesterday."

"A little magic never hurts," I said.

Once home, I cried on the lawn with the sun sinking into the lake that appeared as a long silver blade across the horizon. But this time I was not crying for Mother. I was crying for me. I wanted my life back. I wanted my marriage back. I wanted my own time. But most of all I wanted the suffering for Mother to end. And then, in the midst of my sorrow, hope seeped in like another drug.

I wrestle with my optimism until the Percodan pins my shoulders to the bed.

I found Dad on his hands and knees, pulling small starts of scrub oak out of the garden.

"It's here—" he said as he looked up at me. "It's really here, isn't it?"

I shook my head and sat down beside him. "I don't know.

I think she'll get stronger. It's just so hard to see her in such pain when there's so little we can do."

Dad picked up his pile of seedlings and threw them in a bag. His tears were quickly absorbed into the soil. I moved closer and put my arm through his.

"I thought we would have more time—" he said, "I just thought we would have more time."

"You learn to relinquish," Mother said to me while I rubbed her back.

"You learn to be an open vessel and let life flow through you."

I do not understand.

"It's not that I am giving up," she said, "I am just going with it. It's as if I am moving into another channel of life that lets everything in. Suddenly, there is nothing more to fight."

How can I advocate fighting for life when I am in the tutelage of a woman who is teaching me how to let go?

This evening, August 6, 1986, we celebrated Mimi's eightieth birthday with the entire extended family. A thunderstorm exploded outside. Immediately, we all vacated the living room and sat on the front porch. With our backs against the house, we watched veins of lightning torch the sky.

"It's a dance," Mimi said.

Mother was home alone.

Mother has moved to Mimi and Jack's house.

"Anything to get rid of the monotony," she said.

We sat in the backyard under the sycamore tree, where

the hose was left running to simulate the sound of a stream.

"It's such a healing sound," Mimi said.

Mother rolled up her pantlegs and let the water run over her feet. She bent down gingerly and washed her face.

"Don't tell John I'm playing in the sprinklers," she said. "He'll have me hiking Mount Olympus tomorrow. He's the only person I know who viewed having a hysterectomy as an advantage for backpacking—less weight to carry."

Nothing is working. Mother is writhing in pain.

"Something is terribly wrong," she said after Mimi and I tried to persuade her to eat. "I know my body."

"But the doctor says you are fine. It's just a very slow recovery process," I argued.

In my mind, I don't think she is trying hard enough. She has abandoned the pain medication and relaxation tapes.

In Mother's mind, we are not listening to what she is saying.

For the first time, Mimi is looking like an old woman. She is being worn down like the rest of us. Dad feels like a failure because Mother left home. Mimi and Jack feel like a failure because she is getting worse. I feel like a failure because I am losing my compassion.

We are spent.

I leave tomorrow for a week to participate in an archaeological dig in Boulder, Utah, at Anasazi State Park, sponsored by the museum.

"I'm glad you're leaving," Mother said.

So am I.

MEADOWLARKS

lake level: 4211.00'

A fresh drink of water. A cool breeze. And a swollen Escalante River after a thunderstorm. With the wind billowing my white cotton blouse, I breathe with a clarity of spirit I have not known for months. These expressive skies in constant motion, emotion, move me.

Silence. Juniper green. Cottonwood green. Sage blue. Red earth. Burnished skin. Refuge once again, this time in the reverie of southern Utah.

Behind me is a panel of petroglyphs, three figures etched into the cliff by the Anasazi: a warrior, a woman, and a woman with child. They lived. They died. And something of their spirit remains.

A group of ten high school students and two instructors, of which I am one, have been excavating a site under the supervision of Larry Davis, chief ranger at Anasazi State Park.

Transects are measured, quadrants assigned, and the tedious process of removing top soil begins with small shovels and trowels. Each bit of dirt is screened over a wheelbarrow, potsherds are kept and cataloged, along with fragments of charcoal, bone, and worked stone. The afternoon sun beats down on our backs. We repeat these menial tasks over and over again until it becomes a meditation, of sorts. I am astonished by how much soil we have moved in a day.

The site adjacent to ours has already been excavated. Larry informed us that they had uncovered a burial: an Anasazi woman, approximate date A.D. 1050–1200.

"But what was unusual about this site were the objects we found buried with her—three ollas, corrugated vessels used for carrying water, and several large balls of clay. You could still see the palm prints of the person who had made them." He paused. "She was wearing a turquoise pendant. We believe she was a potter."

"And where is she now?" I asked.

"We reburied her."

I feel like a potter trying to shape my life with the materials at hand. But my creation is internal. My vessel is my body, where I hold a space of healing for those I love. Each day becomes a firing, a further refinement of the potter's process.

I must also learn to hold a space for myself, to not give everything away. It reminds me of the Indian teachings of Samkhya:

> If you consciously hold within yourself three quarters
> of your power and use only one quarter to respond to
> any communication coming from others, you can stop

the automatic, immediate and thoughtless movement outwards, which leaves you with a feeling of emptiness, of having been consumed by life. This stopping of the movement outwards is not self-defense, but rather an effort to have the response come from within, from the deepest part of one's being.

In the middle of Larry Davis's demonstration on primitive technologies, I was handed a pink note by the ranger working at the desk.

"Call home. Brooke."

I got up from the sandstone boulder I was sitting on and felt my legs turn to jelly. It was a long half mile to the telephone.

"Diane's back in the hospital," Brooke said. "It looks like there may be another blockage."

My heart sank.

"Can they operate?" I asked.

"Tomorrow morning," he said. "Is there any way you can get home tonight? Dr. Smith thinks you should be here."

Boulder, Utah, is walled in by wilderness with Lake Powell to the south, Capital Reef to the east, Escalante canyons to the west, and the Boulder Mountains, north. No buses. No trains or planes. No vehicle of my own, just the university van we brought the students in . . .

"I'll find a ride," I said. "I can always hitchhike."

"Just be careful," he said. "I love you."

I hung up the receiver and picked it up again to call the LDS Hospital.

"1–321–1100," I knew it by heart. But the operator couldn't get me through to Mother's room. I put the phone down. I tried to call Dad, no answer. I called Mimi, no answer.

A woman ranger who couldn't help but overhear my conversation said, "I'll find you a ride."

Two hours later, I am in a black, windowless van, sandwiched between two men, one of whom is wearing a cut-off T-shirt which reads, HELMET LAWS SUCK.

"You've got a sick old lady, huh?"

"Yes," I reply, then put on my sunglasses. "I really appreciate the ride."

"No problemo," the dark-haired one answers. "Hope you don't mind if we make a quick stop back at the homestead to pick up a few more folks."

We drive down a dirt road a few miles beyond Boulder until we reach a large white-washed log house. A shredded American flag is flying on a new painted pole. The van stops.

"Enjoy Sculptured Creek . . ." the other long-haired man says.

I sit by the tiny stream and make a bundle of sage. Sculptured Creek is littered with painted tires, iron peace signs, and other abstract metal objects. The men's names are Robert and Mike. They are artists, and we share a common background in our Mormon ancestry, like almost everyone else in the state of Utah.

Robert has just turned forty. Several women helped him celebrate. The long scar that runs up his right arm like a snake is a memento from Vietnam.

"How old are you?" he asks. "Sixteen? You probably never heard of the war."

I am not flattered. "I heard about it . . ."

He and Mike start whistling for someone. It must be a dog. It is a woman. She is running around the house giggling, chased by another man. I look twice—I think she has clothes on.

"What's that one's name?" Robert asks Mike. He shakes his head. They turn to me, "Stay cool, it won't be much longer, we just have to round everybody up."

Seconds later, two women in tube-tops and cutoffs stagger out from behind the bushes with a skinny man holding a shotgun. I can't decide if it's a throwback to Li'l Abner or the 1960s. The man, drunk, opens fire on the pasture.

"I love to make these little fillies run," he shouts as a horse and mule run in circles.

Home appears like a distant mirage in the rural wildness of Garfield County.

Robert and Mike decide I am a dud and ask if I mind riding in the other car. The tie-dyed blonde chooses to ride with them and, as she opens the back of the van, coos, "Oh, another mattress, how sweet!" She falls in face first. Mike slams the door behind her.

I get into the back seat of a lime green Pinto with another man and woman. As we begin to drive away from "the homestead," Robert walks up to the car and motions me to roll down my window.

"It's been a real pleasure, Terry. I hope everything turns out bitchin." He extends his hand.

I reach out to shake it, and he slips me something.

"I wouldn't want one of my girls traveling without protection . . ."

I roll up the window and discover he has handed me a condom. I fight back the tears.

Meanwhile, the couple who are French-kissing behind the steering wheel ask if I mind if we take a detour to look for her lost rock.

"I lost my pink rock with sparkles on it," she says. "I dropped it when I was riding the Harley."

Looking across the sandstoned desert, all I see are pink rocks.

After a good hour of dirt road driving with our heads out the window in search of the dropped rock, she gives up and settles for another.

"It's just not the same," she laments. "I was so attached to the other one."

"I'm sorry," I hear myself saying. "I know how hard it is to lose something you love."

We stop in the town of Scipio for gas, only to find the pumps not working. And who should come swaggering up in his bulging T-shirt and tight-crotched jeans but Robert.

"How'd you like my present?" he asks, trying to pin me against the car with his hips.

"Wrong brand." I remove his hand from my shoulder.

Five hours later, a little after ten, the couple drops me off in front of the hospital. I thank them. We exchange phone numbers. We had become friends. As it turned out, the woman's mother is a textile consultant for us at the museum.

If I had asked enough questions, I am certain I would have discovered Robert and I were related through polygamy several generations back. The dark side of residency.

The family is gathered in Mother's room. Brooke and I check in with our eyes. Lights are low. Mother appears calm, relieved to know there really was something wrong, that the pain wasn't imagined. The operation is scheduled for the morning.

I lean over and kiss her, handing her the bundle of sage wrapped in soft leather.

"I'm so glad you're here . . ." she whispers.

"So am I."

Mother has been in surgery for two and a half hours. Tension is like a shackled horse. Dad is reading. Steve and Grandpa are pacing the halls. I write.

We are pieces of clay being fired again.

One week has passed. Mother and I sit outside, by the hospital fountain and listen to meadowlarks sing, "Salt Lake City is a pretty, little place . . ." It is the song of my childhood. They will be migrating soon.

Mother is frightened, frightened to go on with her life when the future is so uncertain, wondering what her life will be from this point forward.

"I feel like I am on hold until the next thing happens," she says.

She is quiet and frail. She is weary from the physical torment.

"I will not come back here," she says. "I am done with this hospital."

Twenty pounds have been lost. Mother weighs one hundred. But it is her eyes that divulge her suffering. They are deep and dark and distant.

A person with cancer dies in increments, and a part of you slowly dies with them.

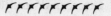

STORM PETREL

lake level: 4210.85'

For ten days, I have done nothing but watch whales quietly surfacing, diving deep, and surfacing.

Brooke and I are in Telegraph Cove, a quaint fishing village at the northern tip of Vancouver Island.

We are assisting Jeff Foott who is making a film on killer whales for Survival Anglia. Yesterday, we were out on Johnstone Strait in a twenty-foot Boston Whaler from six in the morning until nine at night.

I was stationed on a cliff with three biologists who had set up a hydrophone at a depth of fifteen feet in the water to record vocalizations. You hear the whales long before you see them. Even with my untrained ear, I could discern dialects—both by individuals, as well as pods.

Several times, a mother with calves would surface. Sleek black and white bodies wheeling through the sea, their dorsal fins appearing as flags. We listened to their tender murmurings. Some whales passed solitary and silent, while others came into the cove singing.

John Lilly suggests whales are a culture maintained by oral traditions. Stories. The experience of an individual whale is valuable to the survival of its community.

I think of my family stories—Mother's in particular—how much I need them now, how much I will need them later. It has been said when an individual dies, whole worlds die with them.

The same could be said of each passing whale.

We are enshrouded in fog, trolling toward a remote island off Johnstone Strait. A storm petrel led us here. We followed her through the mist until she disappeared. Perhaps she was an apparition.

An orange mask flashes on the cliff face. It is a pictograph with huge ominous eyebrows above open eyes and a gaping mouth. Reflections dance across the water, below the face.

Brooke and I jump off the boat and tie the Whaler to barnacle-encrusted boulders. It is low tide and the hissing of intertidal creatures reminds us we are not alone. We step carefully over kelp-covered rocks on to the lush island.

Spruce, hemlock, and giant cedars humble us. The dense undergrowth of alders and devil's club muffles our voices. It is cool and damp. Little light penetrates this ancient forest.

We walk single file for an hour or more. Suddenly, Brooke stops. At the base of a sheer granite wall are broken cedar boxes.

Three boxes. Three skulls. Inside one box are bones; a partial skeleton with crossed femurs wrapped in a woven mat made of cedar.

One skull is grimacing inside a small cavern beneath the cliff. And still another is wide-eyed staring with its detached jaw from the other twisted box. The bones are disintegrating faster than the textiles that hold them. Rope fragments scatter the clearing like small snakes.

Kwakiutl. These are the old ways of a Northwest Coast Indian people, to hang the dead in burial boxes of cedar over a cliff or suspended from a tree.

We do not stay long, nor do we disturb what we see.

Instead, we walk briskly back to the boat. Looking over my shoulder in the wake of the whaler, one would never know bones, human bones, were hidden in the heart of this island.

I feel like I am floating in salt water, completely at the mercy of currents. Mimi was operated on this morning for breast cancer, September 8, 1986, my birthday.

I accompanied Mimi and Jack to the doctor's for the biopsy report.

"Mrs. Tempest," the doctor said. "I have some good news and bad news. The bad news is the biopsy was malignant. You have a rare form of breast cancer known as Paget's Disease. The good news is at this stage, it is 90 percent curable."

The three of us sat across from his desk, numb.

"I recommend a simple mastectomy. It's an easy procedure, basically like cutting off a mole . . ."

Mimi leaned forward and put her elbows on his desk. "Young man, my breast is no mole."

He blinked. He became flustered.

"Of course not, Mrs. Tempest, I simply meant to say . . ."

"I know what you meant," she interrupted. "And I just want you to know what I mean. I may be eighty, but I am still a woman."

Today, I watched two orderlies wheel her out of surgery

on a stainless steel gurney. I followed them back to the room. They left and I closed the door.

"Damn," Mimi said as she covered her face with her hand.

Mother and I retreated to the lake for the afternoon and sat on a newly constructed dike. The beach had long since disappeared.

We did not discuss Mimi. Instead, we took off our shoes and dangled our feet in the water. I dipped my finger for a taste. I expected salt, it was fresh.

"Thirty-one years . . ." Mother said, smiling. "Happy birthday, dear."

She handed me a present wrapped in white paper with a turquoise ribbon. I unwrapped it carefully and opened the box. Inside was a round glass paperweight with gold and black swirls against a jade background.

I cradled the small globe of waves in my hands.

I remember Mimi asking me as a child to make a lens by curling my fingers around to my thumb. I closed one eye and, with the other, looked through my hand lens. I played with scale. Blades of grass were transformed into trees, a gravel bed became a boulder field. Small rivulets pouring over moss became the great rivers of our continent. My world was my own creation.

It still is.

Now if I take this lens and focus on Great Salt Lake, I see waves rolling in one after another: my mother, my grandmother, myself. I am adrift with no anchor to hold me in place.

A few months ago, this would have frightened me. Today, it does not.

Refuge

I am slowly, painfully discovering that my refuge is not found in my mother, my grandmother, or even the birds of Bear River. My refuge exists in my capacity to love. If I can learn to love death then I can begin to find refuge in change.

ʄʄʄʄʄʄʄʄ

GREATER YELLOWLEGS

ʄʄʄʄʄʄʄʄ

lake level: 4210.80'

"Put aside any romantic or spiritual notions of ancient desert people," said Kevin Jones, an archaeologist, as we walked out to Floating Island in the middle of the salt flats. "Believe me, there was no romance in people's lives ten thousand years ago. They pretty much acted as we would—assessing their situation and making decisions based on the choices at hand."

We hiked up the hill to the cave. Floating Island is an isolated outcrop of limestone separated from the Silver Island Range by at least a mile of salt flats. The cave measures ten meters across its mouth, twelve meters deep. It looks south over the West Desert with Great Salt Lake lapping east. No archaeological excavation has been conducted at this site until now.

The Silver Island Expedition, a project funded by the National Science Foundation, hopes to secure archaeological data and specimens before the West Desert Pumping Project floods the sites.

Excavation of Floating Island Cave was undertaken in order to mitigate the adverse effects of construction work on the island. W. W. Clyde, a Utah-based company, is cutting into the flanks of the island, using it as riprap for the building of the dikes.

Kevin empties a bucket of dirt from the cave on the swinging tray of the quadruped. My job is to screen the debris. I pick out a jasper chip and place it in a vial. I delight over the "tink" of rock in plastic.

I empty another bucket of dirt on the tray and shake it back and forth over the screen. I catalog objects in my mind: twigs, pinyon nuts and hulls, a horned lizard's crown, cedar berries, beads, bone beads; hundreds of tiny bones—femurs, tibias, fibulas, ulnas, scapulas, jaws, skulls (most likely from bats, small rodents, and rabbits); beetle carapaces, grasses, seeds, saltbush leaves, red flakes of jasper and obsidian, basket-pressed stone pottery, animal and human coprolites and dust. Lots of dust. My pores quickly become black.

A small arrowhead rolls back and forth across the screen. Kevin identifies it as a Rose Spring notched point.

I take a break and enter the cave to see what's going on.

Think about a people who made clay figurines with shuttered eyes, and then think about the Fremont, desert people who inhabited the eastern Great Basin and western Colorado Plateau from approximately 650 to 1250 A.D., roughly a thousand years ago. They planted corn, irrigated their fields, and used wild foods with ingenuity. In many ways, the Fremont correspond to the Anasazi to the south. But in many ways, they do not.

The Anasazi were a group of people attached to the Colorado Plateau with a complex social organization: clans, elaborate kivas, and road systems. In contrast, the Fremont were small bands of people, much more closely tied to their immediate environment. They were flexible, adaptive, and diverse.

Some archaeologists believe the Fremont developed from existing groups of hunters and gatherers of this region. They varied from large sedentary populations, villages, to highly mobile clans. An austere rock shelter above the salt flats, a verdant marsh on the edge of Great Salt Lake, and aspen hillsides in central Utah—all house the spirit of the Fremont.

Floating Island Cave looks out over Great Salt Lake. A deeply layered dry cave site helps archaeologists to interpret Fremont groups in two important ways. First, deposits at the sites represent repeated visits by hunting and gathering groups from more than ten thousand years ago to less than fifty years ago. The layer-by-layer excavation of these caves allows us to see how the Fremont developed from underlying hunting and gathering peoples, what their technologies were, and how they evolved. It also shows that although subsistence patterns varied with each cave, together they represent the mobile end of a wide range of subsistence and settlement patterns practiced by the Fremont.

The numerous caves in the limestone mountains of the Great Basin provided natural shelters and storage facilities for the hunter-gatherers who inhabited this region. The Fremont probably visited such caves as Danger, Hogup, Promontory, and Fish Springs in the late fall and winter. Most of these sites were located near spring-fed marshes, which provided edible bulrush runners in winter. Their diet was supplemented by stored foods such as pine nuts collected in the summer and early fall. Other cave sites such as Floating Island and Lakeside were visited for short periods of time where the Fremont collected pickleweed and grasshoppers.

"Hungry?" David Madsen, state archaeologist and director of the excavation, hands me some pickleweed seeds from the small bushes that hug the salt flats.

I taste them.

"Better these than grasshoppers," he says. "Two years ago, we were excavating Lakeside Cave on the western shore of Great Salt Lake when we discovered tens of thousands of grasshopper fragments within the deposits. Bits of insects pervaded every stratum we uncovered. We estimated that the cave contained remains from as many as five million grasshoppers. At first, we had no ready explanation for this phenomenon. Nor could we explain why the cave deposits were so evenly layered with sand from the nearby beach. Some two dozen specimens of dried human feces gave us our first clue: most consisted of grasshopper parts in a heavy matrix of sand. This told us that people ate the hoppers and suggested that the sand was somehow involved in processing them for consumption."

Kevin dumps two buckets of sediment on each of our trays. We continued screening as Madsen continued his discourse.

"Then, last year, practically by accident, we found enormous numbers of grasshoppers that had either flown or been blown into the salt water and had subsequently been washed up on shore, leaving neat windrows of salted, sun–dried grasshoppers stretched for miles along the beach. As a result of varying wave action, as many as five separate rows existed in places. They ranged from an inch wide to more than six feet wide and nine inches thick, and contained anywhere from five hundred to ten thousand grasshoppers per foot. The rows, well sorted by the waves, contained virtually nothing but hoppers coated with a thin veneer of sand."

"That's remarkable," I say as I place more bones in plastic vials.

"But what's interesting," he adds, "is up until then we had envisioned grasshopper collecting to be a tedious task. Now we realize that the hunter-gatherers at Lakeside Cave could have simply scooped up grasshoppers piled along the beaches and consumed them directly."

"And how do they taste?"

"Like desert lobster."

These sites along Bear River Bay with their artifacts reveal that the people were not strictly dependent upon corn. They thrived on the rich resources of the wetlands surrounding Great Salt Lake. Molluscs, fish, waterfowl, muskrats, antelope, deer, and bison, were taken as food. The fibers of bulrushes, cattails, and milkweed were woven into baskets and clothing.

From eight hundred to twelve hundred years ago and, again, from three hundred to five hundred years past, Fremont life flourished on the edges of Great Salt Lake.

The Fremont oscillated with the lake levels. As Great Salt Lake rose, they retreated. As the lake retreated, they were drawn back. Theirs was not a fixed society like ours. They followed the expanding and receding shorelines. It was the ebb and flow of their lives.

In many ways, the Fremont had more options than we have. What do we do when faced with a rising Great Salt Lake? Pump it west. What did the Fremont do? Move. They accommodated change where, so often, we are immobilized by it.

I wonder how, among the Fremont, mothers and daughters shared their world. Did they walk side by side along the lake edge? What stories did they tell while weaving strips of bulrush into baskets? How did daughters bury their mothers and exercise their grief? What were the secret rituals of women? I feel certain they must have been tied to birds.

I return to my screening chores. Hoist another bucket on to the tray, empty it, and spread the sediments. The sands blown across Lake Bonneville ten thousand years ago are now blowing across my hands. I keep screening the strata: bones, tufa, sheep and pack-rat scat, a grass fragment here and there. I put them in vials, put the vials in sacks, the sacks in boxes, and the boxes in the back of the truck, which will transport them to the basement of the Utah Historical Society. It is our uncanny ability to catalog and interpolate, pigeonhole and store our past. Each day in the field translates to one month in the lab.

"Why do you do this, David?" I ask as we pack the pickup.

"Because I want to know how these people coped with the fluctuations. What attracts me to Great Basin archaeology is putting all the pieces together, the complexity of the parts creating the whole. Artifacts alone have never interested me. It's the stratigraphy that speaks. The human stories are told within the layers of sediments."

He turns around, okays the truck, and returns to the trench inside Danger Cave. A shaft of afternoon light strikes the column of sediments. The definitions are stunning.

"You're looking at almost continual habitation in this cave for the last ten thousand years," he says, still profiling the lake gravels. "And the Fremont story is an unfinished one."

Driving back to camp, he elaborates, "During the fifteen

hundred years that the Fremont can be distinguished, they produced an archaeological record as rich, yet as enigmatic, as any in the world. The record of how they lived, reacted, and responded to the changing world around them is a mirror of ourselves—of all peoples at all times in all places."

I look out the window at this seemingly bleak landscape wondering what it means to be human in arid country.

A blast on the salt flats startles me.

"They're preparing for the dikes," Madsen says.

Settled in camp. Solar-heated showers were taken and fresh clothes put on. We hardly recognized one another as we "dressed for dinner."

"We've got an hour before supper," Kevin said, saddling an all-terrain vehicle. "I want to show you something."

I threw my left leg over the black leather seat and put my arms around his waist. Before I could blink, we were speeding up a dirt road in Silver Reef Canyon.

"This is not the best way to see birds," I screamed in his ear.

"We're not here to see birds," he yelled back.

We flew over a hill and bounced on sand. We drove a mile or two further on a seldom-used road with junipers on either side. All I could see in front of me was Kevin's back. He turned off the motor and got off the vehicle.

"Here we are . . ."

Before us was a fleet of plywood tanks, each with a flag painted on the side: Japan, Britain, Russia, and France. In the case of Germany, a swastika decorated the one-dimensional machine.

"What in the world are these?" I asked, walking around each one. "This is like an army theater, and we're miles from anywhere . . ."

"Military targets." Kevin answered while throwing rocks at them. "We found them by accident the other day when we were looking for cave sites."

Horned larks fluttered around the tanks.

"They probably nest inside," I said.

We toyed with the idea of moving the tanks down canyon, marching single file toward camp, but decided against it.

"How long do you suppose they have been here?"

"No idea. But if you look straight up, that's not blue sky you see—that's military airspace. Tomorrow count how many sonic booms you hear."

The crew is back on the road to Floating Island.

Last night the temperatures dropped below freezing, not unusual for mid-October in the Basin. We are blowing into our hands to warm them. It is an orange sky in a purple landscape. Great Salt Lake has advanced since yesterday. The salt flats are on fire, ablaze with morning light.

Rock wrens pierce the silence as we hike up to the cave.

Yesterday the crew uncovered some cordage. Kevin says today we should be able to excavate deep enough to see if it leads to anything. The artifact appears to be circular.

The slow, tedious work continues.

By midafternoon, David Zeanah whisks away the last sediments from the cordage with his brush and uncovers a bird's foot. He follows the string to another leg. He gently lifts it out of the site.

"A bird-foot necklace?" I ask.

The two legs, maybe four inches long severed at the hypotarsus, dangle from the circle. The reticulation on the legs mirrors the twisting of the cordage. Holes have been drilled at the top, with the sinew drawn through and wrapped twice around them. The feet and toes are long and slender, pointing down.

I look at the necklace more closely. My guess: greater yellowlegs, a common transient to Great Salt Lake as they pass southward in the autumn and northward in the spring—an elegant shorebird.

I imagine this necklace being worn in a spring ritual by a clan of bird people to celebrate the fecundity of the marshes.

"Can't you see them dancing around the fire?" I say to Kevin, "dressed in feathers with the shrill cry of bone whistles in the air?"

Kevin rolls back his eyes. "And where are these feathered robes and bone whistles now?"

That night before dinner, I'm helping Jimmy Kirkman, the cook.

"What do you think about the bird-foot necklace?" I ask him.

"I think secretly everyone wants to try it on, but nobody dares to admit their fantasies."

"Unprofessional?" I ask.

"Against an archaeologist's religion," he replies. "It's science, not art."

We both look at each other and immediately have the same idea. We sneak into the supply tent, grab a box of plastic forks and dental floss and together make twelve bird-foot necklaces. Twisted cordage is replaced by spearmint-flavored floss. Where shorebird's legs hung, white forks dangle. We hide them inside my pack.

Dinner is served: linguini with clam sauce. A bonfire is built with wood brought from home. We all move our lawn chairs closer in. Jimmy throws a handful of his magic dust igniting purple and turquoise flames, careful not to reveal his recipe of copper sulphite. I stare at the seductive flames through a kaleidoscope someone has brought, while a strange brew of "archaeologist's cider" is passed around in a well-seasoned gin bottle. Madsen begins telling stories. His gestures become larger. More logs are placed on the fire. More magic dust. Flames rise.

Jimmy winks at me and together we present each archaeologist with their own bird-foot necklace.

Without hesitation, they rip off their coats, put the necklaces over their heads and dance. They dance wildly like tribesmen around the fire, singing songs I have never heard before.

I returned to the museum directly from the field. One of the security guards asked me if I had been to a picnic.

"No, why?" I asked.

"I thought that's why you might be wearing forks around your neck?"

"Oh, these . . ." I replied, looking down at my bird-foot necklace. "New-wave jewelry."

Thousands of objects associated with Fremont culture are cataloged in the museum's collection. We preserve the past for the future. Contact with the artifacts is restricted: white cotton gloves and lab coats, dim lighting, cool room temperatures. Each artifact is numbered. Site recognition is immediate. Any object can be recalled and detailed on the museum's computerized data base known as MIMS (museum inventory management system). It is a controlled environment.

But sometimes the objects run away with you. They seize your imagination and begin to sing songs of another day, when bone whistles called blue-winged teals down to the wetlands of Bear River. You hear them. You turn around. You are alone. Suddenly, the single mitten made of deer hide moves and you see a cold hand shivering inside Promontory Cave. It waves from the distance of a thousand years.

Artifacts are alive. Each has a voice. They remind us what it means to be human—that it is our nature to survive, to create works of beauty, to be resourceful, to be attentive to the world we live in. A necklace of olivella shells worn by a Fremont man or woman celebrates our instinctive desire for adornment, even power and prestige. A polished stone ball, incised bones, and stone tablets court the mysteries of private lives, communal lives, lives rooted in ritual and ceremony.

And sometimes you recognize images from your own experience. I recall looking at a Great Salt Lake gray variant potsherd. A design had been pecked on its surface. It was infinitely familiar, and then it came to me—shorebirds standing in water, long-legged birds, the dazzling light from the lake reflected on feathers. This was a picture I had seen a thousand times on the shores of Great Salt Lake: godwits, curlews, avocets, and stilts—birds the Fremont knew well.

One night, a full moon watched over me like a mother. In the blue light of the Basin, I saw a petroglyph on a large boulder. It was a spiral. I placed the tip of my finger on the center and began tracing the coil around and around. It spun off the rock. My finger kept circling the land, the lake, the sky. The spiral became larger and larger until it became a halo of stars in the night sky above

Stansbury Island. A meteor flashed and as quickly disappeared. The waves continued to hiss and retreat, hiss and retreat.

In the West Desert of the Great Basin, I was not alone.

CANADA GEESE

lake level: 4210.95'

Seventeen monks dressed in white robes were singing vespers before dusk. Mother and I sat inside the Abbey of Our Lady of the Holy Trinity on wooden pews. The light was translucent, the music transcendent. The English translation of what they were singing was "Bring me back home." It was as though we were inside the chamber of a shell. As the chants took on the monotony of waves, we bowed our heads in supplication.

After the vespers, we walked beneath the canopy of cottonwoods that lined the country lane. They were golden. An autumn breeze blew the leaves around us. Mother slipped her arm through mine. She was weak and increasingly fragile. Dressed in a midcalf denim skirt and blouse, with a tweed jacket draped over her shoulders, she was quietly walking with the present. I knew she was tired. I also knew the power of this October afternoon. In another time, this moment would surface and carry me over rugged terrain. It would become one reservoir of strength.

I saw in Mother's face the mature beauty that a woman in her fifties has earned. I also recognized her weight loss not so much as disease, but as a shedding of that which was no longer necessary. She was letting go. So was I. The only clue I had of her pain was in the forthrightness of her voice.

"I used to think the life of a monk was a selfish life," she said. "I don't believe that anymore."

We find a grassy knoll to sit on, as several flocks of Canada geese graze in an amber meadow. Acres of sunflowers bloom against a blue sky. Great Salt Lake, only a few miles west of the Huntsville Monastery, is visible through the corridor of Ogden Canyon.

Small families of geese congregate before their migration. The shadows of clouds crossing over the fields bring them in and out of light.

"Wild geese are my favorite birds," Mother says. "They seem to know where they are from and where they are going."

One can think of migration as merely a mechanical movement from point A to point B, and back to point A, explain it in purely physiological terms: in the fall, the photoperiod is lessened, it correlates with a drop in temperature. Food becomes scarce. Birds eat more. They overeat, put on fat, become restless, and along comes an environmental cue, such as wind, a change in barometric pressure, a cold front—and a rush of flight! Birds migrate.

Alongside the biological facts, could migration be an ancestral memory, an archetype that dreams birds thousands of miles to their homeland? A highly refined intelligence that emerges as intuition, the only true guide in life? Could it be that a family of Canada geese journey south not out of a genetic predisposition, but out of a desire for a shared vision of a species? They travel in flocks as they position themselves in an inverted V formation, the white feathers that separate their black rumps from their tails appear as a crescent moon, reminding them once again that they are participating in another cycle.

We usually recognize a beginning. Endings are more difficult to detect. Most often, they are realized only after reflection. Silence. We are seldom conscious when silence begins—it is only afterward that we realize what we have been a part of. In the night journeys of Canada geese, it is the silence that propels them.

Thomas Merton writes, "Silence is the strength of our interior life. . . . If we fill our lives with silence, then we will live in hope."

Mother and I break bread for the geese. We leave small offerings throughout the meadow. It is bread made by the monks from stone-ground grain. She puts her arm back through mine as we walk shoulder-high in sunflowers.

BALD EAGLES

Rooted. Brooke and I have moved to Emigration Canyon Road, right smack on the trail that Brigham Young and the Latter-day Saints walked down on their way into the Salt Lake Valley.

We planted four Colorado blue spruces today. Housewarming gifts from Mother and Dad. I held the root ball of each tree and blessed them in this supple soil (so unusual for a wintry day), that they might become the guardians of our home.

Dad and Brooke waited impatiently as they leaned on their shovels.

"I'm sorry, Brooke." Dad said. "All this hocus-pocus did not come from me."

I looked at my father as I stood up and clapped the dirt from my hands. "Who are you kidding, Dad? You are the man who taught us as children about divining for water with sticks, taking us out to a job where you had hired a man as a waterwitch to find where a well might be dug."

"Come on, Terry."

"The way I look at it, John," Brooke said. "We're never going to figure it all out, so we might as well acknowledge the intangibles. Who knows, maybe these trees do have souls."

Mormon religion has roots firmly planted in a magical worldview. Divining rods, seer stones, astrology, and visions were all part of the experience of the founding Prophet, Joseph Smith.

Dowsing was viewed negatively by some clergymen, "not because it leads to treasure, but because it leads to information."

Divining rods were understood by many to be instruments of revelation, used not just to locate veins of water or minerals, but to shepherd answers to questions. In folk magic, a nod up meant yes, a lack of movement meant no. Joseph Smith was not only familiar with this tradition, he and his family were practitioners of it—along with use of seer stones, which they used for treasure seeking.

Critics of Mormonism have used this to cast doubt on the origins and faith of this American religion. They dismiss Joseph Smith's discovery of "the golden plates" buried near Palmyra, New York—which contained the holy doctrine translated in the Book of Mormon—as simply an extension of the treasure-hunting days of his youth.

Others claim that Smith's sensitivity to matters of the occult heightened his shamanistic gifts and contributed to his developing spirituality.

For me, it renders my religion human. I love knowing that Joseph Smith was a mystic who ascribed magical properties to animals and married his wives according to the astrological "mansions of the moon."

To acknowledge that which we cannot see, to give definition to that which we do not know, to create divine order out of chaos, is the religious dance.

I have been raised in a culture that believes in personal revelation, that it is not something buried and lost with ancient prophets of the Old Testament. In the early days of the Mormon Church, authority was found within the individual, not outside.

In 1971, when Mother was diagnosed with breast cancer, the doctors said she had less than a 20 percent chance of surviving two years. Mother did not know this. Dad did. I found out only because I overheard the conversation between my father and the doctors.

Months passed. Mother was healing. It was stake conference, a regional gathering of church members that meets four times a year. My father was a member of the stake high council, a group of high priests who direct the membership on both organizational and spiritual matters. President Thomas S. Monson, one of the Twelve Apostles, directly beneath the Prophet, who at that time was Joseph Fielding Smith, was conducting interviews for the position of stake president.

Before conference, President Monson met with my father privately, as he did with all councilmen. He asked him, if called, would he serve as stake president? My father's reply was no. In a religion that believes all leadership positions are decided by God, this was an unorthodox response.

"Brother Tempest, would you like to explain?"

My father simply said it would be inappropriate to spend time away from his wife when she had so little time left.

President Monson stood and said, "You are a man whose priorities are intact."

After conference, my father was returning to his car. He heard his name called, ignored it at first, until he heard it for a second time. He turned to find President Monson, who put his hand on Dad's shoulder.

"Brother Tempest, I feel compelled to tell you your wife will be well for many years to come. I would like to invite you and your family to kneel together in the privacy of your home at noon on Thursday. The Brethren will be meeting in the holy chambers of the Temple, where we will enter your wife's name among those to be healed."

Back home, our family was seated around the dinner table. Dad was late. Mother was furious. I'll never forget the look on his face when he opened the door. He walked over to Mother and held her tightly in his arms. He wept.

"What's happened, John?" Mother asked.

That Thursday, my brothers and I came home from school to pray. We knelt in the living room together as a family. No words were uttered. But in the quiet of that room, I felt the presence of angels.

"What would you have me know?" I asked. "Faith," my great-grandmother Vilate said to me. Mother and my grandmother Lettie and I were helping to pack up her apartment. She was moving herself to a retirement center. "Faith, my child. It is the first and sweetest principle of the gospel."

At the time, I did not appreciate her answer. Faith, to a college coed, was a denouncement of knowledge, a passive act more akin to resignation than resolve.

"Where would faith in the Vietnam War have gotten us? Or faith in the preservation of endangered species without legislation?" I argued.

"My darling, faith without works is dead."

That is all I remember of our discussion. But, today, the idea of faith returns to me. Faith defies logic and propels us beyond hope because it is not attached to our desires. Faith is the centerpiece of a connected life. It allows us to live by the grace of invisible strands. It is a belief in a wisdom superior to our own. Faith becomes a teacher in the absence of fact.

The four trees we planted will grow in the absence of my mother. Faith holds their roots, the roots I can no longer see.

"I can't believe this is my body," Mother said, as she looked in the mirror of the dressing room at Nordstrom's. "I could never have imagined myself this thin . . . and these scars . . ." She shuddered.

I took the red suede chemise, size 6, off the padded hanger and handed it to her. She stepped into the dress and put one arm in, then the other, then buttoned the front and turned the collar up.

"It's perfect, isn't it?" she said, turning sideways to see how it hung in the back.

"Perfect," I replied. "You look absolutely beautiful."

She turned to me, her eyes radiant. "Right now, at this moment, I can honestly tell you, I feel wonderful! John will love this, even if it is extravagant."

She gave me back the dress. "I'll take it," she said, quickly putting on her black skirt and sweater. I held her emerald green jacket behind her as she slipped her arms through.

"Thank you," she said as she picked up her purse. "Shall we move on to our Christmas list?"

The rest of the day was spent in a shopping frenzy: three Christian Dior nightgowns for aunts; a shirt and tie for Steve; a reindeer sweater for Brooke; books for Dan; guitar strings for Hank; a ceramic crèche for Ann; a silver vase for a niece; pistachios for neighbors; a dozen narcissus bulbs; a pair of black patent-leather pumps to go with her new red dress; and two Madame Alexander dolls for her grand-daughters, Callie and Sara.

Waiting for all the packages to be wrapped—she stood while I sat. Mother's energy and quick pace was back. I followed three steps behind.

We had lunch at Hotel Utah: poached salmon. We laughed and chatted over absolute trivia.

"Let's make this an annual affair," Mother said.

We both believed it.

By the time we picked up our packages, it was late afternoon. I drove her home. As she got out of the car, she screamed, "Oh, Terry, look!"

The sun was a scarlet ball shimmering above the lake. Mother put down her shopping bags and applauded.

"How much should I tell her?" Dr. Smith asked me in his office. Mother was in the examining room.

"Tell her the truth," I said. "As you have always done." I could feel the tears well up in my eyes. I was trying to be brave.

"You can't be surprised, Terry. I thought you had accepted this last summer."

"We did. I mean I had, but hope can be more powerful and deceptive than love."

"Her weight loss of eight more pounds is not a result of flu. It's the cancer. She doesn't have much time," he said. He walked out and opened the door to Mother's room.

After the examination, he came back out and said things looked better than he thought, that the tumor he had felt in June was gone, and that the others felt smaller.

Mother was very quiet. On the way home, I asked, "What do you think?"

"It doesn't really matter, does it?" she said. "Let's just take one day at a time."

I had the sense that she wanted to cry. And I thought of her mother, how once in the nursing home, after we had been crying together, I said, "Oh, Grandmother, doesn't it feel good to cry?" and she replied, "Only if you know there is an end to your tears."

Mother and I returned to my new house in the canyon. I fixed some chamomile tea.

"This tastes so good," she said with her hands cupped around the mug. "I can't seem to keep warm."

Mother asked for some more tea. We both settled on the couch. I gave her a mohair shawl to wrap around her shoulders.

"I think I have denied having cancer for years. It's a survival skill. You put it out of your mind and you get on with your life." She paused. "I mean, you have momentary flashes of what is real in periods of crisis and you face them, but then your mind seems to leap over the illness. You forget you were ever sick, much less that you are living with a life-threatening disease. The curious thing in all of this is that I have never acknowledged my anger over losing my breast as a young woman. Isn't that strange? Why would that come up now, after almost sixteen years? I'm angry, Terry."

Mother broke down. We both cried.

"I guess I'm giving up all sense of who I am," she said. "Last month, when John and I were at the beach in Laguna, all I could do was stare out at the waves."

The lake is frozen. Because of the ice, you can travel further west—if you dare.

My friend Roz Newmark and I drove out to the Bird Refuge in my trustworthy station wagon—as far as we could, until the lake stopped us.

It was a dreamscape where the will of the land overtakes you. I felt as though we were standing under the wing of a great blue heron.

As we walked, each step brought about a wheezing from the ice. The ice was thin, showing asphalt below. Off the road, it was a magnifying glass for objects arrested in motion. A floating feather—when was it caught in the clamps of ice? The quill tapered off, bleeding into darkness.

The ice became thinner and thinner, until each step of our boots sounded like vertebrae popping. We stopped. Beneath the icy veneer was a stream of suspended detritus: two snail shells, root fragments and reeds, a Canada goose feather, down, burrs, a piece of styrofoam, a small hollowed corn cob, pebbles, decaying insects, fish bones, carp scales, a woman's shoe.

Farther out, the ice looked solid. It was milky and dense. Roz and I dared each other to go first. Finally, we took hold of each other's gloved hands and began skating away from the road. I held my breath, as though it would make us lighter.

We lasted until moans, groans, and squeaks of the ice sent us back in a hurry. Roz, a dancer by profession, had an enormous advantage as she threw her head back, swung her arms in the air and leaped across the ice. I settled for short shuffles. Back on the road, we swung each other Western-style, joyous in our bravado.

We wandered a mile or two west, still on the same road. Two ravens flew across, their caws like chatter in a cathedral. The quiet returned. Twelve bald eagles stood on the ice of Great Salt Lake, looking like white-hooded monks. From November through March, they grace northern Utah. When the ice disappears, so do they.

Eagles on ice, cleaning up carp: beak to flesh. Flesh to bone. They whittle carrion down to a sculpture, exhibited in a bleak and lonely landscape.

Ice can immobilize, but on Great Salt Lake it creates habitat. I pluck the edge of the ice—it rings with the character of crystal. Ice that supports eagles is of finest quality.

Where the Bear River bends and flows south, the eagles flew. They appeared as small thoughts against the Wasatch Range.

Roz was sitting on her heels, wondering how life goes on in the river beneath the ice. Taking off her gloves, she ran her hand back and forth across its surface. Trapped bubbles, resembling clusters of fish eggs, were a reminder that fish swam below.

"It is comforting to know this," she said.

Mother was dead. I sat up startled and leaned against the pine headboard of our bed. Mother was alive. I wrapped my arms around myself to stop shaking from the nightmare.

But the feeling I could not purge from my soul was that without a mother, one no longer has the luxury of being a child.

I have never felt so alone.

December 16, 1986. Mother and I made a pact that we would no longer discuss how she was feeling physically, unless she wanted to.

"Good," she said. "So what do you have going on today?"

"Grading papers for my class on 'Women and Nature,' at the university," I said. "And I've got a few things to take care of at the museum. What about you?"

"John and I have the annual Church Christmas Ball at Hotel Utah, tonight."

"Are you excited about going?" I asked.

"Very."

"Your red dress?"

"My red dress," she answered.

I saw Mother asking my father to dance before anyone dared step onto the parquet floor.

RED=SHAFTED FLICKER

lake level: 4211.15'

This morning, a red-shafted flicker hammers above the window, offering me a wake-up call. The flicker peers through the glass. I delight in the red flash of feathers on his cheek.

Later, I hear another sound. A backhoe. I open the sliding glass doors and watch the shovel's silver jaw rip into the Earth. Mother Earth. Another house is to be built. I see them digging my mother's grave.

I ring the doorbell. No one comes. The doors are locked. I know Mother is home. I walk to the neighbors and borrow their key. I open the front door. Mother is sitting on the stairs, her hands cradling her head between her knees.

"Are you all right, Mother?" I ask.

She slowly lifts her head. "I am too weak to get to the door."

She starts to sob. I hold her as we rock back and forth on the stairwell.

Another gray day. Fierce winds continue to pull the temperatures down.

Mother gives in. Dad and I take her to Dr. Smith's office. Walking down the long corridor of the medical building, I realize how much I hate this place. The smells, the color of the paint, the wallpaper, the claustrophobia of rooms with no windows. It is 1983. It is 1984. It is June, July, and August, 1986. It is Christmas.

Dr. Smith leads us into the back room, where he carefully inserts an IV into Mother's arm. The air of illness suffocates me. I am nauseous.

For the next two hours, as glucose drips into Mother's veins (to give her strength through Christmas), Dr. Smith unfolds the truth to her like a red rose: petal by petal, he tells her of her limited time, that she is within weeks of her death.

"You mean I have cancer?" she asks.

Dad and I look at each other in disbelief. Dr. Smith looks to us, then to Mother. He takes her hand and gently outlines what she can expect.

Mother's expression is stoic. She looks at Dad, whose tears stream down his cheeks.

"I heard the words but was incapable of internalizing them," Mother said once we were home. "I only saw John's face and could feel what was being said through him."

Tonight we gathered as a family and grieved openly.

"I want it all out by tomorrow so we can enjoy Christmas Eve," Mother said.

Dad and I rolled back our eyes at the woman who must be in control. It was funny. We remain true to our character even in death.

We each spoke of our love for Mother, and she gently said, "I am sorry I cannot be with your feelings. It is very different for me." She did not elaborate.

Steve spoke about being children in 1971, how we would set the timer every fifteen minutes to pray for her to be well.

Dan told of Dad's ritual of always asking Mother to "fix me"—which meant tucking in his shirt before he zipped up his pants.

I recalled a time when I was eight years old: I came home from school, devastated because friends on the playground were making fun of my naturally curly hair when straight hair was in. They called me a "witch." Mother took me by the hand into the bathroom and sat me in front of the mirror.

"Tell me what you see," she said.

I couldn't look.

She took her hand and lifted my chin. "Tell me what you see."

I looked in the mirror, and she said, "I see a beautiful girl with green eyes. I want you to stay here until you see her too."

Dad told the story of being in Hawaii in 1973 with the family. "I don't even remember what we were arguing about but, suddenly, Diane stood up in the middle of the restaurant, pulled the tablecloth off the table and said, 'That's it! I am no longer your slave! From now on, I'm doing what pleases me!' That was the beginning of women's liberation in this family."

Hank sat on the hearth next to me, the fire massaging our backs. I thought to myself, here is the child who, since memory, has lived with the fear that his mother may die. He could not speak.

Dad gave Mother a blessing, to which she added—as the men in the family gathered around her to place their hands on her head—"Someday, I hope Terry and Ann and my granddaughters will be able to stand in the circle . . ." We held hands as Dad spoke of our desire to help Mother through this—that this was our time to care for her as she had cared for us.

"Help us to not be afraid," Dad prayed.

Afterward, he placed his hands on her sculptured face, kissed her, and said, "Diane, we can do this. And I want you to be home. No more hospitals, sweetheart, just home."

Mother strikes a match and lights a white candle in the middle of the pine boughs on the glass table in the living room. She wears her blue satin robe with stars. It is Christmas Eve. We sit in a circle, each holding a silver cup of cranberry juice. Brooke has prepared a toast:

> Last week, Steve and Ann hosted the family Christmas party. It was so natural that what was almost imperceptible was the fact that a new generation had volunteered to make the leap from guest to host. The torch has been passed. This party symbolized the beginning of the changing of the guard.
>
> What are we guarding?
>
> We are guarding the moments given to each of us as members of a family, small bits of time where the family becomes not just a mirror, but a clear, still pond, which each of us can gaze into for glimpses of our real being.
>
> We are guarding the very ideal of family, the bond, the web connecting us all, which gives rise to an energy,

a lust for life lost to those for whom family has lost significance.

We are guarding the buffer of protection that a family's love gives to each of its members, unconditionally, a magic covering that we can wear as armor but not notice its weight.

Let us toast twice. First, to the older generation: May your days come to be many, full of comfort and understanding. May they be spent knowing that those days past have held a completeness uncommon and unknown to many, and that every detail of your beings continues in the lives of those who follow.

To the younger: May we accept these gifts, knowing that they are of this tradition, of this old-fashioned courage, of ethics, and that they can be carried along forever like rusting relics or they can be worn as wings.

Let us wear them as wings.

We raised our cups and drank. Gifts were exchanged among the extended family. Four generations. The presents were opened one at a time.

We arrived for Christmas brunch. Mother greeted us in the foyer. The dining-room table was set as it had always been on Christmas morning: the white damask tablecloth; the Spode dishes, each plate with a tin candleholder from Mexico clipped to its side holding a small red candle; the sterling; the crystal; and a centerpiece of poinsettias and pine boughs.

The naïveté or self-centeredness of children did not recognize this gesture as heroic. There are those things in life that tradition allows you to count on. Of course, we would have Christmas brunch and, of course, Mother would prepare it.

We stood in the buffet line, each of us dishing the traditional food on to our plates: egg and sausage casserole, fresh fruit cocktail, and warbread—a raisin cake passed down by Mamie Comstock Tempest, my great-grandmother, who made this for her family when provisions were scarce during World War I.

We seated ourselves around the table. Everything appeared normal—knives and forks ticking on china, platters of food being passed, more water being poured—until one by one, we noticed Mother was not eating.

I watched her look at Dad, who squeezed her hand under the table. This was the last thing my mother had to do.

DARK=EYED JUNCO

lake level: 4211.20'

Since Christmas we have traveled a thousand miles.

Mother is in bed. I have just come from the kitchen after putting a drop of opium tincture into a glass of water. She drinks the age-old potion for pain.

What does pain prepare us for? Emily Dickinson says, "Pain prepares us for peace."

Thump!

A bird has hit the bedroom window as I write in my journal. I quietly get up from the chaise, open the door, and find a junco stunned on the snow. Its white outer tail feathers are splayed. I want to hold the bird, to bring it inside and save it. But I don't. Instead, I smooth its tiny feathers behind its neck, close the door, and return to Mother.

"What I have learned through all this," Mother says, "is that you just pick yourself up and go on."

I rub her back while she talks.

"I have fought for so long and I have worked so hard to live through this summer, this fall, Christmas—and every minute has been worth it. And now, it feels good to give in. I am ready to go."

"Terry, you have accepted this, haven't you?"

"My soul has—but my mind has not."

A few hours later, Mother hands me a slip of paper, handwritten on both sides.

"I want you to call Dr. Smith with this list of questions, so I know what to expect. I didn't hear a thing the day we were in his office."

I read down the list. "How long is the process of starvation? What happens? Is there pain? Do I force myself to keep eating when nothing stays down? What about liquids? Does that help stay dehydration? What about the opium? Should I continue to take one drop three times a day? Is there anything that will quell the nausea and make me feel more comfortable? Do we need a nurse?"

I call Gary Smith at home with Mother's questions. We go through them systematically, one by one. After about an hour, I return to Mother's bedside.

"Tell me everything," she says.

Suddenly, my clinical self with notebook in hand dissolves.

It is New Year's Eve. Instead of talking about resolutions we wish to make, we are talking about funeral arrangements we must plan. Mother is in the next room, breathing.

Hank thinks our discussion is a betrayal. "I want nothing to do with it," he says. "She is alive."

Dad is becoming increasingly tense, pacing around the family room, unable to make decisions.

I suggest some ideas.

"If you think you have all the answers, Terry, then why don't you just go ahead and plan the whole thing," he snaps.

Dad's fuse is getting shorter as his fears become greater. He disappears into the bedroom.

Steve and Dan agree to choose the plot and casket. Ann offers to make a burial dress.

Dad returns after checking on Mother. "She is asleep. See what you think. I think she could go tonight."

The only light in the room is from the hallway. One by one, we enter, kiss her good-night, then leave.

It is 1987.

Dad closes the door and sleeps next to her.

I hate to go to sleep tonight, knowing another day has passed. At least it has snowed. Finally, the edges of this winter have softened.

None of us are sleeping. Steve and I anticipate the phone call from Dad. Dad cannot sleep, fearing that Mother will die. Dan and Hank cannot sleep because the house is unnaturally still.

The Soleri chimes on our porch keep ringing in the wind. Another storm is brewing.

We wait. We wait for Mother to die. The laziness of grief has us moving slowly.

Each day, I make a decision to dress colorfully: reds, purples, and blues, something to entertain Mother.

This morning she says softly, "You are changing my scenery. I appreciate you dressing up for me. I look forward to your costumes."

It continues to snow. Mother continues to weaken. Somehow, having the world soft and white makes this easier to bear.

Mother has not eaten for weeks. I look into her dark eyes, which widen each day as they retreat farther into her skull.

Nothing seems real. The family is insulated from the outside world by the walls of this house. It feels holy. Friends and neighbors are respecting Mother's privacy.

"This is my death," I can hear Mother say, "nobody else's. It belongs to me in the intimacy of my family."

My days are immersed in the pragmatic details of care. And I love caring for her, we all do, even though there are times when horror splashes our skin like scalding water as we watch her writhe with nausea and pain.

And the other side, always the other side, is as tender as the pain is severe—bathing her, washing her hair, rubbing her body with fine French creams, feeding her ice chips, stroking her hair, her hands, and her forehead.

It is sacred time.

Mother's voice still speaks with her spirited and inquisitive nature. These things don't change. Life in the face of death is merely compressed into grist.

This afternoon, Dan and I came into Mother's room while she was watching Julia Child prepare a chicken dish on television.

"Oh," she sighed with rapt attention. "I would have loved to have tried that . . ."

The household is like a stretched rubber band. Dad left early this morning, angry. He is helpless, unable to save his wife or protect his children. Our calm only fuels his fire.

Mother is increasingly uncomfortable, so weak she can barely stand. I help her onto the scale. Eighty pounds.

"I don't know how to die," she said to me. "My mind won't allow me to rest. You are losing me. I am losing all of you."

It is her restlessness that weighs on me now. Her anguish over us—the living watching the dying,—the dying watching the living. She is still the peacemaker trying to create a calm in the midst of her death. And there is nothing she can do to ameliorate the situation.

"I feel the tensions, Terry."

An individual doesn't get cancer, a family does.

I feel calm, having just returned from a brisk walk along the base of the foothills. The balm of fresh air; Great Salt Lake glistened on the horizon. The valley is in sharp focus, crystal clear. I am reminded that what I adore, admire, and draw from Mother is inherent in the Earth. My mother's spirit can be recalled simply by placing my hands on the black humus of mountains or the lean sands of desert. Her love, her warmth, and her breath, even her arms around me—are the waves, the wind, sunlight, and water.

She is resting. The nurse came and gave her a shot of Demerol. All Mother said today is how much she wants to sleep, "to not think or feel, just sleep."

I never imagined we would walk to the place where what we hoped for was death. Sleep. It is the same thing.

I read Mother a poem this afternoon by Wendell Berry:

THE PEACE OF WILD THINGS

When despair for the world grows in me
and I wake in the night at the least sound
in fear of what my life and my children's lives may be,
I go and lie down where the wood drake
rests in his beauty on the water, and the great heron
feeds.
I come into the peace of wild things
who do not tax their lives with forethought
of grief. I come into the presence of still water.
And I feel above me the day-blind stars
waiting with their light. For a time
I rest in the grace of the world, and am free.

"Read it again," she said. "Slowly."

The rubber band holding the household together snapped. Dad feared he was having a heart attack. I am so anxious, water glasses slip from my hands and break. Every day we think it can't get any worse. But it does. We don't know what to do for Mother.

Dr. Smith is coming up to the house to install a morphine drip, which will take the edge off Mother's pain.

Mother was greatly relieved to see him.

"How are you feeling, Diane?" he asked empathetically. He seemed to know what we couldn't. He sat on the edge of the bed. We gave them their privacy.

A few minutes later, Dr. Smith opened the door and asked for our help. I assisted him as he put an IV just under Mother's clavicle. The blood, our mother's blood, was spurting on the Marimekko sheets. We watched him search for a vein with the needle. Each time he tried, we winced, until the sickle-shaped needle finally hooked skin to tie down the line. Mother's face was strained. As the doctor shot the blood back into her vein she pulled back her neck. It was pale blood, not the deep red I had once seen. Dr. Smith set up the drip, the bag of glucose and morphine on a mechanical tree that held the pump. He showed us how to operate it, how to mix the right formula, the shot of Heparin needed to keep her veins open. I tried it and immediately pricked my finger with the needle while trying to put the cap back on the syringe.

I tried it again and got it right.

In the living room, Dr. Smith told us it was going to get a lot worse before Mother would die. That news seemed unfathomable. He said Mother would be comfortable now, and that he would check in often, whenever we needed him. He took his coat, walked out the door and I faced my father, with no answers.

His eyes were red with rage. His voice pinned me against the wall. "My home will not be turned into a hospital. Enough is enough. I can't take it anymore. It's so easy for you to play Pollyanna and say what a wonderful experience this is, but you don't have to live here. You can go home to Brooke, to the peace of another house and forget what is happening. I can't."

"As soon as Diane lapses into a coma, I'm taking her to the hospital. Someone else can deal with it—by then it won't matter, anyway."

SANDERLINGS

rrrrrrrr

lake level: 4211.35'

"Close the door," Mother said. "I've been waiting for you to get here all morning." She held out her hand. "Something wonderful is happening. I'm so happy. Always remember, it is here, in this moment, and I had it."

I didn't understand.

"Something extraordinary is happening to me. The only way I can describe it to you is that I am moving into a realm of pure feeling. Pure color."

I took off my coat and folded it over the chair. Sitting down beside her, I replied, "Maybe that's what this business of eternal life is . . ."

She took my hand again. "No, no, you're missing it—it's right here, right now . . ."

This afternoon, as I was lying next to Mother, she took hold of my arm.

"Terry, this isn't a joke, is it? I mean is there any possibility?"

"Of what, Mother?"

"Is there any possibility I may not die?"

I paused, not knowing what she was asking or what she wanted to hear.

"I don't think so . . ."

She closed her eyes and sighed. "Ah, I'm so glad."

Ten breaths per minute. The morphine pump purrs. Mother floats. She is relaxed. No more anxious days of nausea and wondering how to die. It is easier on her, harder on us. I miss the conscious edge between acceptance and struggle.

Mother sleeps.

I watch her skeleton push through skin, emerging bone by bone, rib by rib, until her vertebrae have become the ladder my fingers climb as I rub her back. Her face is a death mask, skin stretched over skull. The bone from her ear to her eye is like a bridge, and the orbital structures that protect her eyes look like spectacles. Nothing is hidden. She sees with dark, wide sunken eyes.

Her hands remain unchanged, becoming more beautiful, more expressive each day. Her fingers seem to lengthen and her nails grow long. We hold each other's hands, and I see and feel the years of my mother's nurturing: the hands that cradled me, cuddled me, stroked my head at birth; the hands that bathed me, disciplined me, and combed my hair as a child; the hands that called me, prepared my food, wrote me letters, and loved my father's body; the hands that worked

in the garden on long summer days planting marigolds for
fall.

These hands even at death are beautiful.

Death is no longer what I imagined it to be. Death
is earthy like birth, like sex, full of smells and sounds and
bodily fluids. It is a confluence of evanescence and flesh.

It is so peaceful lying next to Mother. I am not afraid.
We listen to Chopin and talk some. Mother finally says, "I
just want to listen to the silence with you by my side."

The fullness of silence. I am learning what this means.
Mother and I have grown so used to simply being, at times
I find it difficult to speak.

Yesterday she said, "Terry, talk to me about something
. . ." I panicked. I didn't know how to respond. I stood up
and quickly said, "Okay, just a minute, let me get you some
ice chips." While in the kitchen, I leaned against the
counter, my mind throbbing with ideas that I have been
yearning to explore with her, but by the time I returned,
the moment had passed. Words had once again lost their
urgency. Silence. That ringing silence. I sat by the side of
her bed and held her hand while the ice chips melted.

Mother mentioned this morning how much the morphine pump sounds like helicopters coming over the rise.
Her comment stopped me, and then I remembered my own
association with helicopters, the dream I had four years
earlier, when all this began.

Changing the morphine drip frightens me. I draw out 5 cc's of morphine from the amber bottle. It measures 75 milligrams. I could draw out more. Mother watches me. We are both thinking the same thing. I shoot the morphine through the blue target of the 5 percent dextrose bag instead of her vein. Then I draw up 1 cc of Heparin. Inject that into the bag and massage the fluid so it is sufficiently mixed. I puncture the bottom of the bag with the IV apparatus and hang it on the mechanical tree like a hummingbird feeder. I clear the line of air bubbles, then turn off the pump. Next, I clamp the active IV line, pull out the needle from the Heparin lock near Mother's clavicle and insert the new IV. I unwind the old tubing and rethread the new. Turn the pump back on. Reset the monitor and I am finished. After I see all is in order, I tape the Heparin lock to Mother's skin and spiral the white tape around the tubing for security. I have another few hours to relax.

Touch is more important than ever. I notice Mother holds my hand tighter than usual.

"It feels so good to hold your hand," she said. "I don't feel so disconnected."

Steve arrives. We trade places.

After dinner, Dad took the men of the family to the basketball game at the University of Utah. Mother felt like talking.

"What I leave with you, Terry, is this: Follow your feelings. I have followed mine."

I asked her once again if she thought Brooke and I should have a child.

"I would hate to see you miss out on the most beautiful experience life has to offer. What are you afraid of?"

"I am afraid of losing my solitude, my time to retreat and

my time to create. Brooke is as ambivalent as I am. My ideas, Mother, are my children."

"I would rather hold you in my arms than one of your books." She paused.

"You asked my opinion, and I have given it to you."

"And I will follow my feelings."

She rubbed my back. "I love you so. We don't need words, do we? Do you know how wonderful it is to be perfectly honest with your daughter? Do you know how rich you have made my life? I am seeing circles, circles of love."

She took her hand off my back and turned the other way. "I need to be alone, dear."

"Come as soon as you can," Dad said over the telephone. "The night nurse doesn't think she will last the day."

When I arrived, Mother was disoriented, saying she felt like she was off her center, that she didn't know what was happening to her.

"I keep dreaming about elephants and melting ice," she said faintly.

I timed her breaths. Four per minute.

Dad came in. We both held her hands. She closed her eyes. We became incredibly frightened, not knowing if this was it, feeling she might slip away at any moment.

Suddenly, sunlight streamed into the room, striking Mother's face. It was as though God's hands were reaching out to her. And then the light shifted to another part of the room. Her breathing stabilized. Dad left.

Steve, Dan, and Hank entered. I stayed. We began to tease Mother about who was the cutest baby. Mother came alive.

"You all looked the same, little clones. That's why we didn't have any more."

Her laugh, unexpected and free, caught us off guard. We read from a book of local poetry, which a neighbor had sent:

> A sad-eyed dog
>   with tired feet
> stepped out
>   into the busy street
> without a warning
>   he was gone,
> a crumpled heap
>   upon our lawn.

The five of us became hysterical, laughing so hard we were sobbing. Dad ran into the room in a panic. Steve read the poem for a second time and we doubled over in laughter again—this time with Dad crying. In the middle of this bedlam, Mimi walked into the room carrying a tray of barbequed chicken wings. We read it a third time and she had to put the tray down.

The mood of the day was set. Mother was ebullient. We forgot our grief. The doorbell rang. Friends visited. Dr. Krehl Smith walked in. Mother asked him how his trip to Myrtle Beach had been, how his wife, Beverly, was feeling, and so on and so on, until finally he said, "No more of this, I'm onto you. What about Diane?"

"Who?" she asked.

"Diane—you."

"At peace," she said, "and not in pain."

Krehl left. Another dear friend arrived. They talked incessantly. Mother drooled over ward gossip, news from the neighborhood, and current affairs.

"Delicious," Mother said, with a Cheshire cat grin. "I feel like I'm back in the world."

Her friend having held her composure walked out the

front door and broke into tears. Mimi held her, saying, "We all feel that way."

Brooke came in with his ski clothes still on, looking more like a wildman from the north than a son-in-law. He kissed Mother. His cheeks were still cold and red from the windburn.

"I'm glad somebody in this family looks healthy," she said. "Give me your blue eyes and blond hair."

We were exhausted. Mother kept going. "Today has been wonderful," she said, stretching her arms. "I'm so happy. I didn't want the end of my life to become boring."

It is 8:00 P.M. Mother has ordered the family out of her bedroom. She is watching *Gone With The Wind*.

"I will ring the bell you gave me, if I need you."

She was sitting upright with the lights out, her glasses on, and pillows propping her back.

An hour later, she rings the bell. She is lying on her back. I carry another pan of green-black bile that Mother has vomited into the bathroom. As I pour it into the toilet, I throw up, too. It is the stench of death. The movie is still playing. I hear Melanie say on her death bed, "Do not squander time, that is the stuff life is made of."

Mother asked if I noticed a difference in her today. I told her, yes, that she was more restful. I then asked her if she felt any different.

"No," she said. "I don't feel different, but I sense you are all treating me differently."

I count her breaths. They have the intensity and fullness of a surfacing whale's.

A week ago, Mother asked me to write her a story. Today, I read it to her:

A long, long time ago, when stray shells on a beach were as common as gulls, there sat a silver-haired woman on a silver-stained log. Driftwood. You could say they both had become driftwood. And there she sat, staring at the waves.

"Stallions," she thought. "The waves break as stallions."

She rocked back and forth on the log, digging her heels in the sand. She saw seven crows. Black on white. Or was it white on black? She could hardly tell, as the sea foam swirled around the dark forms. They didn't move. Perhaps they were not birds at all, but stones. She knew her eyes could not be trusted. They were clouding over with age. Even so, she would ask the next person to tell her what she had seen.

But no one came.

The old woman stiffened with each gust of sea breeze, and she began to smell of salt. The crows, the stones (she still couldn't be sure), seemed to be moving closer—or she to them. She felt herself tiring and closed her eyes.

She dreamed of the way things are seen, as she continued to rock back and forth on the log, clutching her elbows for warmth.

It was new moon, and the tides were changing. Two men were walking. One remarked to the other how solitary the beach had become. They passed by the woman. They passed by the driftwood. They passed by the birds.

"What is that?" one asked. "Over there—"

He pointed toward the tethered figure on the weathered wood.

"Just crows," the other replied. "Just crows."

And they continued to walk along the edge of the surf without getting their feet wet.

The old woman in her reverie had heard what she hoped might be true.

"Just crows . . ."

And the seven crows she had almost mistaken as stones stayed near her.

"Trust your feelings . . . I have trusted mine." Mother's words echo in my heart.

I get up to wash my hands. In the mirror, I see my mother's face.

January 15, 1987. It is 2:00 P.M. The wind continues. The large bedroom windows rattle with each gust. I fear they will shatter. The house is cold. I am alone with Mother as she is dying. And for the first time in weeks, I am afraid. The child in me, which lives as long as she does, wishes that the doorbell would ring, that Mimi or Grandmother or my aunts or anyone, would be there to help me.

Mother is restless. As she breathes, her throat rattles. Her neck is swollen. I worry that she is uncomfortable. I moisten her lips with a pink sponge swab. She appears to be talking with someone in this room, someone I cannot see. All at once, she rises and says, "I'm ready to go," and begins walking out the door. The morphine pump wavers, ready to tip over, as the morphine line threatens to snap.

I leap to my feet and grab her waist before she collapses on the floor. I lay her gently back on the bed and pull the covers around her. She looks to the corner of the room and points. "Can't you see?"

I look but see nothing.

Mother falls back into a deep sleep, and silence returns to the room.

I am left trembling, frightened by all I don't know, all

I can't see. I leave Mother, close the door, and escape into the living room. Through the windows, my eyes focus on Great Salt Lake. It's still there, mirroring the sky. I collapse under the weight of grief and cry. I curl up on the floor in a fetal position. I am sick of death. I want life. I want to surround myself with flocks of white pelicans in full summer sun. I want to dance naked on sand dunes. I yearn to have someone hold me and save me from this pain.

And then it hits me—I still have a mother. She is in the room next door and deserves to know how I feel, to see the underside of my heart. Dad keeps telling me she no longer understands what we are saying, that she is in a coma. I don't believe him.

I walk back into her room, kneel at her bedside, and with bowed head and folded arms, I sob. I tell her I can no longer be strong in her presence. I tell her how agonizing this has been, how helpless I have felt, how much I hurt for her, for all that she has had to endure. I tell her how much I love her and how desperately I will miss her, that she has not only given me a reverence for life, but a reverence for death.

I cry out from my soul, burying my head in the quilt that covers her.

I feel my mother's hand gently stroking the top of my head.

Five P.M. The doorbell rings. It is Dr. Gary Smith. He walks into the bedroom to check on Mother.

"It's very close," he says. "I'm sorry John isn't here. Please tell him he has done well." He places his hand on Mother's wrist. "Good-night, Diane." He looks around the room, unplugs the telephone near her bed, and, as quickly as he was in, he is out.

Steve and I are getting ready to change the morphine

drip. Our aunt, Ruth, has arrived with a pot of beef stew and is stirring it over the stove in the kitchen. Dan is asleep downstairs. Hank is at work.

Suddenly, Dad roars up the driveway only to find it blocked by cars. His tires screech as he races back down and parks on the street. The door slams. Thundering up the stairs, he yells, "Get out! All of you! This is my house and my wife!"

Ruth leaves immediately, simply saying, "John, your dinner is on the stove."

Dad walks into the bedroom, finds us there and suddenly, the alarm on the pump goes off.

"Beep . . . beep . . . beep . . . beep . . . beep . . ."

It has never done this before. Steve and I look at each other. Mother's eyes are closed.

"I want you out of here, now!" he says. "I'll take care of this."

"Dad, we have a problem here, let's get it under control and then we'll leave." Steve says very rationally.

As our father's rage is unleashed, my brother and I feed him line, plastic tubing to untangle. For twenty minutes, we keep feeding him line. We have less than one hour to fix the malfunction before Mother's veins will close. I pull the IV needle from her clavicle, shoot her with Heparin and return to the pump to figure out what is wrong. All the while, the alarm keeps beeping, flashing its red light into the room.

Lights in the room are flickering as the storm wages its own battle outside. Tempest. Our father is honoring his name.

"Go. Now."

"Just help us untangle the line, Dad. We've almost got it," Steve keeps saying calmly, as we continue threading plastic tubing through his quivering hands. After almost forty minutes, the alarm stops. Silence. The problem is solved.

I hook the IV needle back into Mother's vein. Prepare another 5 cc's of morphine. Steve brings in the bag. I look at my father, whose eyes are like a rabid dog's. Shoot the morphine into the glucose bag, massage it, hang it from the tree, set the gauge, bend down and kiss Mother's forehead. With her eyes closed, she whispers, "Thank you." "I love you." I whisper back. And walk out the door.

Dad follows us to our cars. I look at him but I have no words. It is a blizzard. Driving up the canyon, almost sliding off the road, I harbor my own rage and wonder if the wind will ever stop.

I am home. Our power is out. Brooke is lighting candles. My brothers and I agree we will not return to the house. Our father is the one who needs to be with Mother when she goes.

I understand him, but I don't have to forgive him. Not tonight.

I'm sitting on our chaise longue, sipping tea. This morning a pink light outlined the eastern skyline. The sky is blue. The mountain before me is crisp in detail. All of the wildness of last night is gone.

Mimi and Grandmother called. They let me talk out my feelings. They both said the same thing, "Trust life. Understanding is love."

For years, I have imagined being by Mother's side at the moment of her death. I have to let that go—she has taught me there is no one moment of death. It is a process. Besides, she—

Dad just called—he wants us there . . .

It is the third day since Mother's death. A candle is lit. Let me begin.

Friday, January 16, 1987

Dad called around noon.

"I'm sorry," he said. "I behaved poorly last night. I just wanted to be alone with Diane and I wanted to protect you kids from the burden I was afraid to carry. I realized last night that I cannot save Diane from death or shelter you from seeing it. I realized a relationship is not made in the last thirty days or twenty-four hours, but in a lifetime. And Diane and I have lived well." He paused. "She's going quickly. Please come. I need all of you. I don't want to be alone."

Walking into her room, I could see death was imminent, and I was surprised to see the physical changes from the night before. Her color had changed—especially around the mouth and nose. Her face was waxen. Her feet were cold. It was as though dying moves from your toes upward.

Mother's breathing was regular, but strained as she exhaled. So much going out. So little coming in. I knelt at the foot of her bed with the soles of her feet pressed against my forehead. It was the only place I could feel her pulse. I rubbed her legs under the mohair blanket. They were like ice. Dad paced the room, occasionally sitting next to her to hold her hand. We took turns.

From one until four in the afternoon, we sat near her. A meditation. Her breaths could now be heard as moans. Her eyes were haunting, open, and clear. Time was suspended like watching a fire. Gradually, Mother's breaths became a mantra and the death mask we feared was removed.

Dad spoke of what it had meant to him to "take care of our own." In these hours, we began to realize the magnitude of these past weeks, months, years. Talk of everyday life crept in, basketball scores, the day's news, even laughter, and there, Mother lay dying. I never doubted her presence.

The light in the room deepened. It occurred to me that Mother would wait until after sunset. And it was an exquisite one. An apricot aura radiated above the purple Oquirrh Range. I told Mother what a beautiful sunset it was—I recalled her applause.

We turned a small lamp on. Mother's color looked better and, for a moment, we believed she would never die. The belabored breathing continued. We took turns holding her hands. Rubbing her forehead. Moistening her mouth. And we could feel the cold moving up her body. Her head was turned now, and with each breath her head drew back, reminding me of the swallow I beheld at Bear River, moments before it died.

Dad began to get nervous. He worried that Mother could go on for a few more days, that we had kept vigil too many times. He smiled with an anxious grin, saying, "Diane, you may outlast me yet . . ."

He wanted to be there when she died, and yet he didn't. He was afraid he would not be able to survive it. After a few minutes of wavering, Dad decided to pick up his car downtown. Brooke said he would drive him.

Dan left. Steve and Ann disappeared to other parts of the house. Hank was gone. I was alone with Mother.

Our eyes met. Death eyes. I looked into them, eyes wide with knowledge, unblinking, objective eyes. Eyes detached from the soul. Eyes turned inward. I moved from the chaise across the room and sat cross-legged on the bed next to her. I took her right hand in mine and whispered, "Okay, Mother, let's do it . . ."

I began breathing with her. It began simply as a mirroring of her breath, taking the exertion of her exhale, "ah . . . ," and reflecting back a more peaceful expression, "awe . . ." Mother and I became one. One breathing organism. Everything we had ever shared in our lives manifested itself in this moment, in each breath. Here and now.

I was stunned by the way her eyes fixed on mine—

the duet we were engaged in. At other times, I just closed my eyes and merged with her, whispering once again, "Let go, Mother, let go . . ." But mostly, it was just breath . . . slowing down, quieting down, until only the sweetest, faintest expressions of breath remained.

Steve and Ann walk into the room. They can feel her spirit: Mother's wisps of breath creating an atmosphere of peace.

I feel joy. I feel love. I feel her love for me, for all of us, for her life and her birth, the rebirth of her soul.

I say to Steve, "She's going . . . she's going . . ."

He sits next to her and takes her other hand. Faint breaths. Soft breaths. In my heart I say, "Let go . . . let go . . . follow the light . . ." There is a crescendo of movement, like walking up a pyramid of light. And it is sexual, the concentration of love, of being fully present. Pure feeling. Pure color. I can feel her spirit rising through the top of her head. Her eyes focus on mine with total joy—a fullness that transcends words.

Just then, we hear the garage door open. Dad and Brooke are home. A few more breaths . . . one last breath—Dad walks into the room. Mother turns to him. Their eyes meet. She smiles. And she goes.

He kneels by her side, takes her hand, and says, "Diane, finally you are at peace."

7:56 P.M. I stood by Brooke. I felt as though I had been midwife to my mother's birth.

We knelt around her body. Dan held Mother's head in his lap. Our father offered a prayer for the release of her spirit and gave thanks for her life of courage, of beauty, and for her generosity, which enabled us to be part of her journey. He asked that her love might always be with us, as our love will forever be with her. And with great humility, he acknowledged the power of family.

In the privacy of one another's company, we openly celebrated and grieved Mother's passing. A flock of sanderlings wheeling over the waves of grief.

Erich Fromm writes: "The whole life of the individual is nothing but the process of giving birth to himself; indeed, we should be fully born when we die."

A full moon hung in a starlit sky. It was Mother's face illumined.

BIRDS=OF=PARADISE

lake level: 4211.65'

Mother was buried yesterday.

These days at home have been a meditation as I have scoured sinks and tubs, picked up week-worn clothes, and vacuumed.

I have washed and wiped each dish by hand, dusted tables, even under the feet of figurines.

I notice my mother's hairbrush resting on the counter. Pulling out the nest of short, black hairs, I suddenly remember the birds.

I quietly open the glass doors, walk across the snow and spread the mesh of my mother's hair over the tips of young cottonwood trees—

For the birds—

For their nests—

In the spring.

"Wait here, I want to show you something . . ." My friend, who runs a trading post in Salt Lake City, disappeared into the back room and returned with a pair of moccasins.

They took my breath away. The moccasins were ankle-high and fully beaded, including the soles, which were an intricate design of snakes. Cut glass beads: red, blue, and green, hand-sewn on white deerskin. As I carefully turned them, I wondered how anyone on earth could wear these. To walk in these moccasins would destroy the exquisite handwork.

An Indian woman who had been browsing, smelling the baskets of sweet grass, quietly walked over to the counter.

"Those are burial moccasins," she said. I handed one to her, but she would not touch it. "You won't see many of these."

My friend looked at the woman and then at me. "She's right. A Shoshone woman from Grantsville, ten miles south of Great Salt Lake, brought them in yesterday. They had just buried her grandmother in Skull Valley with the best they had: a buffalo robe, pendleton blankets, jewelry, a beaded dress of buckskin, and the moccasins. The granddaughter made two pairs."

The Indian woman in the trading post identified herself as Cherokee. She explained how, among her people, they sew only one bead on the soles of their burial moccasins.

I thought of the Mormon rituals that surround our dead: the care Mimi and I took in preparing Mother's body with essential oils and perfumes, the way we dressed her in the burial dress Ann had made of white French cotton; the high collar that disguised her weight loss, the delicate tucks from the neck down, the simple elegance of its lines. I recalled the silk stockings; the satin slippers; and the green satin apron, embroidered with leaves, symbolic of Eve and associated with sacred covenants made in the Mormon temple, that we tied around her waist—how it had been hand-sewn by my great-grandmother's sister at the turn of the century. A gift from Mimi. And then I remembered the white veil which framed Mother's face.

I tried to forget my encounter with the mortician in the hallway of the mortuary prior to the dressing, the way he led me down two flights of stairs, through the maze of coffins, and then abruptly drew the maroon velvet curtains that revealed Mother's body, now a carapace, naked, cold, and stiff, on a stainless steel table. Her face had been painted orange. I asked him to remove the make-up. He told me it was not possible, that it would bruise the skin tissues. I told him I wanted it off if I had to remove it myself. The mortician left in disgust and returned with a rag drenched in turpentine. He reluctantly handed me the cloth and for one hour, I wiped my mother's face clean.

I remember arriving at the chapel early, so I could check on the flowers and have some meditative time with Mother's body before the funeral. The face paint was back on. I stood at the side of my mother's casket, enraged at our inability to let the dead be dead. And I wept over the hollowness of our rituals.

The same funeral director put his hand on my shoulder. I turned.

"I'm sorry, Mrs. Williams, she did not pass our inspection. We felt she had to have some color."

"Won't you sit down." he said. "Death is most difficult on the living."

"I'll stand, thank you." I said taking my handkerchief to Mother's face once again.

One by one, family members entered the room, walked to the open coffin and paid their respects. This was the first time my grandmother Lettie had seen her daughter since

Christmas Eve. Confined to a wheelchair in a nursing home, her only contact had been by phone. My grandfather Sanky stood behind her with his hands on her shoulders. She mourned like no other.

As is customary in Mormon tradition, Steve and I brought the white veil down over Mother's face and tied the bow beneath her chin. I had hidden sprigs of forsythia down by her feet. The casket was closed. Dan and Hank placed the large bouquet of tulips, lilacs, roses, and lilies, across the top. Dad stood back, frozen with protocol.

Friends came to call. The line grew longer and longer. We became public greeters, entertaining their sorrow as we put aside our own.

I cannot escape these flashbacks. Some haunt. Some heal.

Today is Mother's birthday. March 7, 1987. She would be fifty-five. I lay one bird-of-paradise across her grave.

In a dugout canoe, Brooke and I paddle through a narrow channel of mangroves. A four-foot tiger heron peers out with golden eyes, more mysterious, perhaps, than any bird I have ever seen. The canal widens and we find ourselves in a salt water bay reminiscent of home.

We are in Rio Lagartos, Mexico.

Row upon row of flamingos are dancing with the current. It is a ballet. The flamingos closest to shore step confidently, heads down as they filter small molluscs, crustaceans, and algae through their bills before the water is expelled through either side. These are not quiet birds.

Behind the feeders, a corp de ballet tiptoes in line, flowing in the opposite direction like a feathered river. They too are nodding their heads, twittering, gliding with the black portion of their bills pointing upward. They move with remarkable syncopation.

American flamingos. Gray. White. Fuchsia and pink.

They span the red spectrum. Feathers float in the water. Delicately. Brooke leans over the gunnels of the canoe and retrieves one. It contracts out of water. He blows it dry.

The birds are a pink brushstroke against the dark green mangroves. A flock flies over us, their necks extended with their long legs trailing behind them. Pure exotica. In the afternoon light, they become flames against a cloudless blue sky. Early taxonomists must have had the same impression: the Latin family name assigned to flamingos is *Phoenicopteridae,* derived from the phoenix, which rose from its ashes to live again.

There is a holy place in the salt desert, where egrets hover like angels. It is a cave near the lake where water bubbles up from inside the earth. I am hidden and saved from the outside world. Leaning against the back wall of the cave, the curve of the rock supports the curve of my spine. I listen:

Drip. Drip-drip. Drip. Drip. Drip-drip.

My skin draws moisture from the rocks as my eyes adjust to the darkness.

Ancient murals of ceremonial art bleed from the cavern walls. Pictographs of waterbirds decorate the interior of the cave. Herons, egrets, and cranes. Tadpoles and serpents stain the walls red. Human figures dance wildly, backs arched, hips thrust forward. A spear-thrower lunges toward fish. Beyond him stands a water-jug maiden faintly painted above ferns. So lucent are these forms on the weeping rocks, they could be smeared without thought.

I kneel at the spring and drink.

This is the secret den of my healing, where I come to whittle down my losses. I carve chevrons, the simple image of birds, on rabbit bones cleaned by eagles. And I sing without the embarrassment of being heard.

The men in my family have migrated south for one year to lay pipe in southern Utah.

My keening is for my family, fractured and displaced.

PINTAILS, MALLARDS, AND TEALS

lake level: 4211.85'

April 1, 1987. Great Salt Lake has peaked for the second time at 4211.85'.

The birds have abandoned the lake. Borders are fluid, not fixed. There is no point even driving out to the Refuge. For now it is ocean. I hardly know where I am.

Since Mother's death, I have been liberated from my optimism. I have nothing to hope for because what I hoped for is gone.

There are no mirages.

A Sunday morning in April. It is General Conference. A gathering of Saints. Mormons from all over the world convene on Temple Square to sit on the wooden pews of the tabernacle (pews stained to look like oak, even though they are pine) to hear the latest counsel and doctrine from the Brethren.

I drive by the cast-iron gates, heading west with the gulls. Red light on North Temple. I stop. With my windows rolled down, I can hear the Tabernacle Choir singing "Abide With Me, 'Tis Eventide," as it is being broadcast throughout the grounds.

Abide: to wait for; to endure without yielding; to bear patiently; to accept without objection; to remain in a stable or fixed state; to continue in a place. "Abide with me," I have sung this song all my life.

Once out at the lake, I am free. Native. Wind and waves are like African drums driving the rhythm home. I am spun, supported, and possessed by the spirit who dwells here. Great Salt Lake is a spiritual magnet that will not let me go. Dogma doesn't hold me. Wildness does. A spiral of emotion. It is ecstacy without adrenaline. My hair is tossed, curls are blown across my face and eyes, much like the whitecaps cresting over waves.

Wind and waves. Wind and waves. The smell of brine is burning in my lungs. I can taste it on my lips. I want more brine, more salt. Wet hands. I lick my fingers, until I am sucking them dry. I close my eyes. The smell and taste combined reminds me of making love in the Basin; flesh slippery with sweat in the heat of the desert. Wind and waves. A sigh and a surge.

I pull away from the lake, pause, and rest easily in the sanctuary of sage.

Ten miles east, General Conference is adjourned.

In Mormon theology, the Holy Trinity is comprised of God the Father, Jesus Christ the Son, and the Holy Ghost. We call this the Godhead.

Where is the Motherbody?

We are far too conciliatory. If we as Mormon women believe in God the Father and in his son, Jesus Christ, it is only logical that a Mother-in-Heaven balances the sacred triangle. I believe the Holy Ghost is female, although she has remained hidden, invisible, deprived of a body, she is the spirit that seeps into our hearts and directs us to the well. The "still, small voice" I was taught to listen to as a child was "the gift of the Holy Ghost." Today I choose to recognize this presence as holy intuition, the gift of the Mother. My prayers no longer bear the "proper" masculine salutation. I include both Father and Mother in Heaven. If we could introduce the Motherbody as a spiritual counterpoint to the Godhead, perhaps our inspiration and devotion would no longer be directed to the stars, but our worship could return to the Earth.

My physical mother is gone. My spiritual mother remains. I am a woman rewriting my genealogy.

On the west shore of the lake, across from Dolphin Island, I cover myself with hot, white sand. Oolitic sands. These sands, perfectly round, have a nucleus of quartz or the fecal pellet of the tiny brine shrimp. An outer shell is then built around the core in concentric layers of aragonite. Great Salt Lake pearls. I wear them. My secret dowry of wealth.

A blank spot on the map translates into empty space, space devoid of people, a wasteland perfect for nerve gas, weteye bombs, and toxic waste.

The army believes that the Great Salt Lake Desert is an ideal place to experiment with biological warfare.

An official from the Atomic Energy Commission had one

comment regarding the desert between St. George, Utah, and Las Vegas, Nevada: "It's a good place to throw used razor blades."

A woman from the Department of Energy, who had mapped the proposed nuclear-waste repository in Lavender Canyon, adjacent to Canyonlands National Park, flew into Moab, Utah, from Washington, D.C., to check her calculations and witness this "blank spot." She was greeted by a local, who drove her directly to the site. Once there, she got out of the vehicle, stared into the vast, redrock wilderness and shook her head slowly, delivering four words:

"I had no idea."

Brooke and I with a few good friends decided to go south for the Fourth of July: Dark Canyon, a remote area in southeastern Utah. On the map it appears without character. For years, I had dreamed of entering this primitive area where one can walk barefoot on slickrock for days, finding cool, midday soaks in hidden potholes. But first, we had to descend into Black Steer Canyon. Dark Canyon was one day away.

Somewhere between thoughts of rattlesnakes and finding the safest route down the steep, talus slope, I lost my footing. Skin, bone to stone, my head hit on rock and with my hands in my pockets I tumbled down the cliff until I was caught and saved by an old, juniper tree.

One of my companions, who was hiking behind me, yelled to see if I was all right. I answered yes, but as soon as I rolled over and tried to stand up with my pack still on, he said, "No, Terry—you're not all right. Lie down."

The river of blood that dyed my white shirt red was not from a nosebleed, but rather a long, deep pressure wound on my forehead, which had popped open like a peach hitting pavement. Lying down on the scree slope, I couldn't get two thoughts out of my mind: How badly am I hurt? And who will take care of me? I could feel myself losing consciousness.

Brooke hiked back up the slope to reach me. Fortunately, one of the members of our group was an emergency medical technician, with a well-supplied first-aid kit. I looked into her eyes as she was trying to stop the bleeding and asked, "Am I going to die?"

"Yes," she said. "But not today."

I relaxed.

"All you need when you get home," one friend teased, "is some long bangs."

We had been joking all morning about how the only good part of this hike down Black Steer Canyon (now christened "Bum Steer Canyon") was that we wouldn't have to climb back out. The good news that I was going to live was now dampened by the view of the cliff before me. I was the only person who could carry me out.

With a tightly bandaged head, after some water and a twenty-minute rest, Brooke and I climbed out of the canyon. Once atop the mesa, where the going was flat, we traversed the desert in hundred-degree heat, pushed on by a shot of energy only adrenaline can produce. It took us four hours to get back to the car.

Ten hours later, we arrived in Salt Lake City and met Brooke's brother-in-law, a plastic surgeon at the LDS Hospital. He reopened the cut, which I saw with a mirror in hand, for the first time. It ran from my widow's peak straight down my forehead across the bridge of my nose down my cheek to the edge of my jaw. I saw the boney plate of my skull. Bedrock.

I have been marked by the desert. The scar meanders down the center of my forehead like a red, clay river. A natural feature on a map. I see the land and myself in context.

A blank spot on the map is an invitation to encounter the natural world, where one's character will be shaped by the landscape. To enter wilderness is to court risk, and risk favors the senses, enabling one to live well.

The landscapes we know and return to become places of solace. We are drawn to them because of the stories they tell, because of the memories they hold, or simply because of the sheer beauty that calls us back again and again.

I will return to Dark Canyon.

The unknown Utah that some see as a home for used razor blades, toxins, and biological warfare, is a landscape of the imagination, a secret we tell to those who will keep it.

"It's no secret among traditional peoples," Mimi said sitting next to me on my bed. "Many native cultures participate in scarification rituals. It's a sign that denotes change. The person who is scarred has undergone some kind of transformation."

The next time I looked into the mirror, I saw a woman with green eyes and a red scar painted down the center of her forehead.

"She had felt labor pains all night long," my cousin Lynne explained. "And then in the middle of the night, she woke up, walked into the bathroom, and gave birth to a tumor. She reached into the toilet bowl, pulled out the bloody mass and set it in the sink. She walked into the kitchen, opened the cupboard, returned with a plastic bag, and placed the tumor inside it, ziplocked it shut, put it in the refrigerator and went back to sleep. The next morning, Mimi called the doctor."

"And what did the doctor say?" I asked.

"The doctor said she would meet her at the hospital for some tests. Mimi arrived with Jack, pulled the plastic bag out of her purse and handed it to the nurse behind the desk. Gary Smith, who was on call at the time, looked at the mass, looked at Mimi and said, 'Mrs. Tempest, I can tell you right now, this is a cancerous growth.' The biopsy later was diagnosed as a mixed müllerian sarcoma."

"When did they perform the hysterectomy?"

"That afternoon," Lynne said.

"And what's the prognosis?"

"It doesn't look good."

"You Americans, why is death always such a surprise to you? Don't you understand the dance and the struggle are the same?"

The voice of a Zimbabwean woman comes back to me. We had met in Kenya a few years back. I had walked out on a film on famine in Ethiopia. I could not bear the suffering. She followed me out, grabbed my arm, and brought me back in.

Same hospital. Same floor. Different room. My legs barely support me. I walk in with a bouquet of miniature roses from our garden. Mimi is sitting up in bed, reading *Omni* magazine.

"I'm home . . ." I say smiling, having just returned from leading a ten-day pack trip into the Tetons sponsored by the museum. Dad had come as a participant.

I handed her the flowers trying to keep up my persona.

"I'm so grateful you and John were away, Terry. I can't bear to put you all through this again. At least they have me down the hall from where Diane was."

We both laughed, then cried.

"Mimi, what happened?"

"I let go of my conditioning . . . I could only say this to you. But when I looked into the water closet and saw what my body had expelled, the first thought that came into my mind was 'Finally, I am rid of the orthodoxy.' My advice to you, dear, is do it consciously."

Consciously? Here is the woman who, at eighty, dragged her two granddaughters to a weekend symposium entitled "The Way of the Dream," where for two days we watched twenty hours of film of Jungian dream analyst Marie-Louise von Franz, lecture on archetypal language. (The second day we showed up in our nightgowns.)

Consciously? Here is the woman who, when I was twelve years old, told me that the dream I had of letting a great horned owl fly into my house and perch on my shoulder was an omen that I would menstruate soon.

Consciously? Here is the woman who had seriously considered taking LSD under the supervision of a medical doctor so she could have "a mind-altering experience," who had read herself straight out of Mormonism and into Eastern religious thought—but refused to replace one dogma with another.

How could she have been more conscious?

And then I looked at this woman I loved, my spiritual mentor, who was a charter member of Greenpeace before I had ever heard of them, who was a financial supporter of every conservation group in America—and then I remembered; she also voted for Ronald Reagan twice.

"What are we going to do?" I asked.

"I promise you, Terry, I am fine. Cancer at eighty is very different from cancer at forty. You must get on with your life and I will get on with mine. We will just go with it."

"We've harnessed the lake!" exclaims Governor Norm Bangerter. "We are finally in control."

One hundred Utah Republicans wave their ceremonial cowboy hats in the air and cheer. These are the party donors known as "The Elephant Club," who are eager to see for themselves the completed West Desert Pumping Station, which will extend millions of acre-feet of water into a salt desert.

David Grant, from the Bureau of Economic Development, explains to the crowd, "The sixty-million-dollar expenditure for this project is an insurance premium. It will benefit the state of Utah in a specific set of circumstances. If Mother Nature goes beserk on us and we have massive flooding—well, that's one set of circumstances the policy won't cover. And if we find ourselves in a drought—the policy wasn't needed. But let me ask how many of us cash in our homeowner's insurance? We're just happy to have it."

The pumping project will return Great Salt Lake to elevation 4208.00'. It aids AMAX, Southern and Union Pacific Railroads, and Great Salt Lake Minerals. There has already been a $240 million loss to railroads, transportation, mineral, wildlife, recreation, and residential interests. The potential loss to the south shore—where the Salt Lake City International Airport, I-80, I-15, and railroads reside— would be close to $1 billion.

Railroads and industry surrounding Great Salt Lake understand—so much so that Great Salt Lake Minerals contributed $200,000.00 to the pumping project study, and Southern Pacific put up $7 million out of its own pocket to help finance the $23 million bid to restore the ten-mile causeway access to the pumps.

I hear my father's voice: "It all comes down to dollars and cents . . ."

AMAX isn't complaining. After the water is diverted from Great Salt Lake to the West Desert, the mineral content increases from 7 to 15 percent because of evaporation. A canal from the holding pond to the magnesium plant has been designed and is one step away from being implemented. AMAX expects increased revenues of $30 million and the creation of two hundred jobs.

The state of Utah may deny subsidizing industry at the taxpayer's expense, but they cannot deny that they are an administration with great imagination. Consider some of the alternatives in state files for managing Great Salt Lake:

University of Utah professor of geology William Lee Stokes advocated nuking the lake, creating a cavern by the atomic explosion that would drain the water to the center of the earth.

Another idea: Dye the lake purple. Certain colors enhance evaporation 10 to 15 percent. Dark purple is one of them. The problem with dying Great Salt Lake purple was not purple pelicans and gulls, but rather that the dye would only penetrate 30 inches of the water's surface. They would have to paint the lake repeatedly and with the volume of water in Great Salt Lake at 30 million acre-feet, this management scheme would have depleted the world's source of purple dye, not to mention a cost of $300 million to taxpayers.

But all is not lost. Utah has itself a major tourist attraction. According to Lt. Governor Val Oveson, "This could become a tourist destination on an international scale—

pumping salt water into a desert—there's nothing like it in the world!"

Public tours are already in motion. Thousands of curious individuals and a fair share of skeptics have boarded buses across the causeway from Lakeside, Utah, to witness the pumps. Public officials believe if they charge a dollar per person, they can recover the state's $60 million with that many tourists.

Ron Ollis, public affairs officer for the division of water resources, who conducted the first half-dozen tours last month, said, "While we were conducting tours, the air force was dropping bombs. The military did maneuvers above the causeway for the public. Some of the pilots stormed the railroad tracks in 'Top Gun' fashion. Everybody loved it."

The Utah Test and Training Range, adjacent to the pumping station, is property of the United States Air Force. The contractor who put the natural-gas line into the station had to sign a document absolving the air force of liability in the event that his workers hit a mine or a fused bomb.

When you enter the project you are given a pair of Decidamp hearing protectors. You squeeze-roll them between your fingers, put them in your ears, and wait for them to expand.

The world is silenced.

In the pumping station everything is explained:

AIR COMPRESSOR, 300 KW GENERATORS, NATURAL-GAS LINE, AIR CLUTCH, RIGHT ANGLE GEAR DRIVE, ENGINE COOLANT LINE, HEAT EXCHANGES, ENGINE COOLANT SURG TANK.

A banner over the engine reads, DRESSER-RAND NATURAL GAS-FUELED ENGINE, BUILT WITH PRIDE IN PAINTED POST, NEW YORK. THREE OF THESE ENGINES WILL DRIVE INGERSOLL-RAND FIFTY-FOOT-TALL PUMPS THAT WILL DROP THE LEVEL OF GREAT SALT LAKE BY 1,300,000 GALLONS PER MINUTE FOR THE DE-PARTMENT OF WATER RESOURCES OF UTAH.

I hold on to the railing to see the pump shaft below. It resembles the beater in my mixmaster.

Outside, I take off my ear plugs and put them in my skirt pocket. Salt foam swirls beneath the bridge. Phalaropes spin near shore. The four-mile canal that shuttles Great Salt Lake to the desert has been named "Rio Buena Vista," after the mythical river that the Spaniards supposed drained the salt lake into the Pacific Ocean.

"How long will these pumps last, given the corrosive effect of the salt?" I ask Ollis.

"The pumps are made of aluminum-bronze alloy. They have a fifty-year life expectancy."

"How much does it take to operate these pumps?"

"$2.3 million per year. The $100,000 per month needed to pay for the natural gas that fuels the pumps is included in the $60 million appropriated by the state legislature."

"And how long will it take for the lake to go down with the pumps operating?"

"We anticipate a drop of one foot the first year, that's 2.2 million acre-feet of water displaced—or 325,000 acres or 500 square miles of water in the West Desert, depending on how you choose to look at it. Keep in mind, right now there are 30.2 million acre-feet of water in Great Salt Lake, roughly 2400 square miles."

Ron Ollis is sharp. I like him.

Governor Bangerter addresses the Elephant Club: "This was the kind of decision you wish you didn't have to make, but when the lake is lapping at your doorstep, you do what you have to do to solve the problem. And let me tell you, Great Salt Lake is a big problem."

The Governor cuts the red ribbon. There is a round of cheers. The West Desert Pumping Station is officially christened. One of the Elephant Club members turns to Great Salt Lake before getting back on to the bus. "Now, what I'd really like to see us do is pump the salt out of the lake completely."

I sit on the banks of the new "Rio Buena Vista" and watch a vein of Great Salt Lake flow west. A rattlesnake stretched across a boulder stops my eyes. The head and rattles have been cut off by a trophy hunter. I walk over to the snake and lift its body, which still articulates between each delicate rib. Forty-two diamonds run down its back. It must measure over three feet long. I wrap the snake around my neck, leave the pumping station, and set out across the desert.

Poet Robert Hass writes, "You hear pain singing in the nerves of things; it is not a song."

My father no longer hunts. Neither do my brothers.

"I can no longer participate in the killing," Dad said. "When I see the deer, I see Diane."

Hank put his gun down years ago. So did Dan. Steve carries his rifle into the hills, but he has not shot a deer since 1983.

"I see the buck in my scope but I can't find a good enough reason to pull the trigger."

For the men in my family, their grief has become their compassion.

This afternoon, I walked along the shores of Farmington Bay. Four California gulls, three pintails, a blue-winged teal, one Canada goose, two mallards, a western grebe, and an American merganser—dead—individual birds, randomly shot. Their limp bodies were strewn along the beach.

I realize months afterward that my grief is much larger than I could ever have imagined. The headless snake without its rattles, the slaughtered birds, even the pumped lake and the flooded desert, become extensions of my family. Grief dares us to love once more.

BITTERNS

lake level: 4210.20'

I found the birds! Malheur National Wildlife Refuge in southeastern Oregon, has adopted and absorbed the flocks of Great Salt Lake. Not all of them, of course. But many. Especially the colony-nesters. Thousands of white-faced ibises, double-crested cormorants, and snowy egrets circle the lake. Huge cumulus clouds looking like clipper ships sail across the sky. The air is quivering with pintails, mallards, and teals. It is like coming home.

Bitterns stand their ground in the camouflage of cattails, their bills pointing toward heaven. A short-eared owl flaps over fields that are back-lit in pink. Even curlews are dancing on the uplands. These are my wetlands that sparkle and sing. It has been so long since my lungs have been filled with the musky scent of the marsh.

I sit on the rich, moist earth, green earth and draw my knees to my chest. All is not lost. The birds have simply moved on. They give me the courage to do the same.

These wetlands held in the spacious arms of the Great Basin are refuges—Malheur in Oregon; Stillwater and the Ruby Marshes in Nevada; Fish Springs and Bear River in Utah; sapphires in the desert bordered by birds.

ΓΓΓΓΓΓΓΓΓ

SNOWY PLOVERS

ΓΓΓΓΓΓΓΓΓ

lake level: 4209.10'

The day the pumps were turned on, the lake did an about-face on its own. Great Salt Lake is receding, having dropped more than two feet from last year's lake level high of 4211.85'.

Where the water has pulled back, the land looks as though it is recovering from a long illness. Barbed-wire fences act as strainers. Sheets of algae and rotting vegetation hang like handmade paper and bobs of tangled hair.

A "bomb catcher" is being built in the West Desert. It is the newest component of the West Desert Pumping Project.

The United States Air Force has disclosed information from their own environmental assessment report: although most bombs exploded on impact during training missions conducted since World War II, some did not. There is a fear that unexploded bombs, including some in watertight containers embedded in the salt flats, might be dislodged by the pond water and float toward Great Salt Lake.

"Imagine a giant comb about eleven hundred feet long," says Brent S. Bingham, president of Bingham Engineering, Inc., the Salt Lake City company that has designed the bomb catcher. "It consists of twenty-two hundred fiberglass bars, five feet tall and six inches apart, that will span the spillway, preventing bombs from being carried into the lake by the stream of water pouring out of the new holding pond west of the Newfoundland Mountains."

Mr. Bingham told newpaper reporters today that no bombs have been seen floating in the pond, which is two and a half to three feet deep, but state officials don't want to take any chances.

Dee Hansen, Director of the Utah Department of Natural Resources says, "The bomb catcher is not for major bombs. It's for phosphorous bombs and different types of bombs in canvas bags. . . . The Air Force experimented with a bunch of stuff out there. Most of it has probably deteriorated if it didn't explode. But the Air Force is pretty cautious, and we want them to be." He adds, "An explosive ordnance disposal unit from Hill Air Force Base inspected the corridor for the twelve-mile-long Newfoundland Dike before construction began. They found some unexploded ordnance in the area, which were retrieved."

All I can see are thousands upon thousands of tumbleweeds cartwheeling over the surface of the water, beating the floating bombs to the strainer.

The West Desert Pumping Project is one of thirteen engineering efforts nominated for the 1988 Outstanding Civil Engineering Achievement Award presented by the American Society of Civil Engineers.

"The award recognizes engineering projects that demonstrate the greatest engineering skills and represent the greatest contribution to civil engineering progress and mankind," said Sheila Brand, spokesperson for the society.

We had several calls at the museum today from people who wanted to know if there had been an earthquake. According to the seismology station on campus, there had been no tremors.

It turns out the rattling vibrations were in the air, not the ground.

Atmospheric shock waves were generated when the air force exploded twenty-five thousand pounds of munitions near Great Salt Lake at 2:30 P.M.

Airman First Class Jay Joerz, with Hill Air Force Base public affairs, said, "Munitions are disposed of on a regular basis at the test and training range just west of the lake. Weather conditions must have been just right for the shock wave to carry so far. Yesterday we had another twenty-five thousand–pound explosion and nobody noticed."

Snowy plovers have shown a 50 percent decline in abundance on the California, Oregon, and Washington coasts since the 1960s, due to the loss of coastal habitats. The National Audubon Society petitioned the U.S. Fish and Wildlife Service in March 1988 to list the coastal population of the western snowy plover as a threatened species. The present population estimate for the western United States, excluding Utah, is ten thousand adult snowy plovers, rising to thirteen thousand individuals after breeding season. A knowledge of inland population numbers and distribution is essential to our understanding of the status of the species as a whole. That's why we are counting them in Utah.

I have been combing the salt flats north of Crocodile Mountain for them since early morning. So far, my count is zero.

Margy Halpin, a non-game biologist leading the survey for the Utah Division of Wildlife Resources, and I are walking parallel to each other, maybe a half-mile apart. The distance between us feels greater than it is because of the intense heat and glare of the alkaline terrain.

I walk slowly, following the western shoreline of Great Salt Lake. Clay bluffs along the water's edge resemble Normandy: they have eroded into fantastic shapes, alcoves, and tunnels from past wave action. There are no footprints here.

Windrows of brine flies and ladybug carcasses twist along the beach. Otherwise, it is littered with limestone chips, which clamor like coins when walked upon. The heat is brutal. I pause to dip my scarf in the lake and tie it back around my forehead.

I turn west away from the lake and walk back across the salt flats. Another hour passes. I see movement. Two snowy plovers skitter ahead. Margy also has them in view—we motion each other simultaneously waving with our right hands. If they were not dashing across the white-brocaded landscape, they would be impossible to see. They are perfectly camouflaged.

Margy and I join each other and sit on the salt to watch them. I have to squint through my binoculars to shut out the light reflecting off the flats. Heat waves blur the plovers.

They appear to be foraging on half-inch golden beetles. We pick up one of the insects close to us for a better examination of what the plovers are eating. The golden carapace is translucent, gemlike. We set the creature back on its course, and it skeeters away.

Snowy plovers are the scribes of the salt flats. Their tracks are cursive writing, cabalistic messages for the bird-watcher who cares enough to follow their eccentric wanderings.

We spot two more adult plovers with chicks. Two chicks. Margy and I check with each other to make sure.

"Ku-wheet! Ku-wheet! Ku-wheet!"

On this day, their calls are the only dialogue in the desert.

The snowy plover is considered to be an uncommon summer resident around the shores of Great Salt Lake, so our total count of six on June 11, 1988, is no surprise. They are listed as common residents of Pyramid Lake in Nevada and Mono Lake in California. Long-term distribution records show that snowy plover populations rise as Great Salt Lake retreats. More habitat supports more birds.

What intrigues me about these tiny white birds with brown bands across their breasts is how they manage their lives in such a forbidding landscape. The only shade on the salt flats is the shadow they cast. There is little fresh water, if any. And their diet consists of insects indigenous to alkaline habitats—brine flies and beetles.

Fred Ryser explains, in *Birds of the Great Basin,* how this "wet food, even during the driest and hottest time of year, contains much water of succulence . . . with each mouthful of food, the plover drinks."

To cool off, the snowy plover stands in the salt water and lets the brackish water evaporate from its body.

Another question rises with the heat of the salt desert. Why don't their eggs bake?

Snowy plovers nest in shallow scrapes, open and exposed. Some plovers will use brine fly pupal carcasses for a nesting bed, and then line them with small pebbles and shells. Both male and female snowys incubate the eggs; on hot days, such as today, they trade places frequently, alternating from sitting to standing (not so unlike us). Parenting plovers have been seen to soak in salt water and, upon returning to their clutch of eggs, will ruffle their wet feathers, sprinkling the eggs with water. An average clutch size is three eggs. Research suggests half the broods in Utah might fledge two young.

Margy and I share drinks from her canteen. I have a throbbing headache, which tells me I have been ignoring my own need for water. I fear I may be suffering from heatstroke and begin to worry about getting home. Too much exposure.

Before walking back through shoulder-high greasewood, I take a quick swim in the lake. The silky waters of Great Salt Lake cool my parched skin, even though the salt burns. This offers a momentary reprieve from my nausea. I lick my swollen lips and am careful not to rub my eyes.

I catch up with Margy and follow her through the maze of greasewood. We hear rattles and stop. It is the driest sound on earth. We take another path and walk briskly toward Crocodile Mountain.

Driving home alone on the solitary dirt road that winds around the lake, I am struck with delirium. I stop the car. Nothing looks familiar. I get out and heave violently behind the sagebrush.

The next thing I remember is waking up in a dark motel room in Tremonton, Utah. I call Brooke to see if he can tell me what happened. He is not home. Snowy plovers come to mind. They can teach me how to survive.

November 15, 1988. Lettie Romney Dixon passed away at noon from lingering illness. My grandfather, Sanky, has not left her side for months. Last night, I sat with them all night long. He held her hand and I held his. Mother felt near. Death has become a familiar landscape. I can smell it.

We prepare my grandmother's body. Her tiny arms stiff around her chest are like chicken wings because of Parkinson's Disease. They have not been able to hold those she loved for years. This was the pain I could not embrace. Her blue eyes did. And now they are closed.

My uncle Don, from out of town, walks into the room. We hug. I see my mother's face in his and do not hear a word he says.

Once home, I split open a ripe pomegranate. Red juice trickles over my hand and spills on to my lap as I eat the tart, succulent seeds.

Mothers. Daughters. Granddaughters. The myth of Demeter and Persephone lives through us.

"This cannot be a coincidence, can it?" I ask my cousin Lynne, over the telephone. "Three women in one family unrelated by blood, all contract cancer within months of each other?"

"I have no idea, Terry. All I know is that my mother has breast cancer and her surgery is tomorrow."

"Is there a pattern here, Lynne, that we are not seeing?"

Lynne's voice breaks. "What I do know," she says, "is that I resent so much being asked of the women and so little being asked of the men." There is a long pause. "I'm scared, Terry. I'm scared for you and me."

"So am I. So am I."

Something is wrong and I can't figure it out—the egg collection at the Museum of Natural History. On first appearance, these clutches of eggs arranged in a nest of cotton move me. The size range and color differentiation is stunning, from the pink and brown splotching of a peregrine falcon's eggs to the perfectly white, perfectly round eggs of a great horned owl. And the smaller birds' eggs are individual works of art, canvases on calcium spheres—some spotted, some striped.

But when I hold one of these eggs, there is no gravity in my hand. A weightless shell. Life has literally been blown out through a pinhole.

It dawns on me, eggs are not meant to be seen. This collection is a sacrilege, the exposed medicine bundles of a tribe. These eggs are the hidden wealth of a species, tenderly guarded beneath the warm, bare brood patch of a female bird.

Secrets were housed inside these shells, enough avian lives to repopulate a marsh, even Bear River. But we have sacrificed them in the name of biology to substantiate the obvious, that we know where each bird comes from. These hollow eggs are our stockpile of evidence.

On my way home, I drop by to visit Mimi. She is painting on her easel in the dining room. She rinses her brushes and we sit in her turquoise study.

"What's on your mind?" she asks.

"Tell me what eggs symbolize?"

She runs her hand through her short gray hair. "For me, it is where life originates. In mythic times, the Cosmic Egg was believed to be held within the pelvis of the ancient Bird Goddess. Why do you ask?"

I describe my encounter with the egg collection at the museum, how disturbing it was.

"The hollow eggs translated into hollow wombs. The

Earth is not well and neither are we. I saw the health of the planet as our own."

Mimi listened intently. She stood and turned sideways to switch on the lamp. It was dusk. I could not help but notice her distended belly, pregnant with tumor.

"It's all related," she said. "I feel certain."

"The total number of snowy plovers counted around Great Salt Lake was 487, with 26 young in 11 broods," I tell Mimi as we drive out to Stansbury Island. "Biologists figure we may have two thousand breeding pairs in Utah." She wanted to get out of the house for a change of view. Her strength is holding in spite of the cancer.

We had just seen four snowys scurrying between clumps of pickleweed.

Just outside Grantsville, thousands of Wilson's phalaropes and eared grebes were feeding in the median ponds adjacent to the freeway. No doubt a migratory stop.

In recognition of Great Salt Lake's critical role as a migrational mirror reflecting ducks, geese, swans, and shorebirds down for food and rest, the Western Hemisphere Shorebird Reserve Network has identified the lake as a crucial link in the chain of primary migratory, breeding, and wintering sites along the great shorebird flyways that extend from the arctic to the southern tip of South America.

By becoming part of the network, Great Salt Lake could gain international support for local conservation efforts and wetlands management. It has been nominated by the Utah Division of Wildlife Resources, the U.S. Fish and Wildlife Service, and Bureau of Land Management. And just recently, the Utah Division of Parks and Recreation, along with the Division of State Lands and Forestry, endorsed the nomination.

To qualify, a site must entertain in excess of 250,000 birds a year, or more than 30 percent of a species' flyway population.

Great Salt Lake qualifies. It hosts millions of birds in a season. Don Paul points out, however, that the lake qualifies on the basis of Wilson's phalaropes alone—flocks of 500,000 to 1,000,000 are not uncommon during July and August, when they are en route to South America.

The Western Hemisphere Reserve Shorebird Network has paired Great Salt Lake with Laguna Del Mar Chiquita, the salt lake in the Cordoba region of Argentina where the phalaropes winter. They are sister reserves.

"Think about one phalarope flying those distances," Mimi said, looking through her binoculars. "And then think about flocks of phalaropes, millions of individuals being driven on their collective journey. We go about our lives giving little thought, if any, to such miracles."

There is a chorus of wings navigating the planet. Twenty million shorebirds migrate through the United States each year to arctic breeding grounds in the spring and back to their wintering sites in South America. One bird may cover as many as fifteen thousand miles in a year.

Great Salt Lake is a refuge for these migrants. And there are certainly other strategic sites along the migratory path, essential to the health and well-being of those birds dependent upon wetlands. The Copper River Delta in Alaska, Canada's Bay of Fundy, Grays Harbor in Washington, the Cheyenne Bottoms of Kansas, and Delaware Bay in New Jersey are just a few of the oases that nurture hundreds of thousands of shorebirds.

Without these places of refuge, successful migrations would cease for millions of birds. None of these sites are secure. Conservation laws are only as strong as the people who support them. We look away and they are in danger of being overturned, compromised, and weakened.

Wetlands have a long history of being dredged, drained, and filled, or regarded as wastelands on the periphery of our towns. Already in Utah, there are those who envision a salt-free Great Salt Lake. A proposal has been drafted for the Utah State Legislature to introduce the concept of "Lake Wasatch." The Lake Wasatch Coalition would impound freshwater flowing into Great Salt Lake from the Bear, Weber, Ogden, and Jordan Rivers and other tributaries, by means of more than eighteen miles of inter-island dikes stretching through four counties between Interstate-80, Antelope Island, Fremont Island, and Promontory Point.

They see Lake Wasatch as fifty-two miles long and twelve and a half miles wide—three times the size of Lake Powell in southern Utah and northwest Arizona.

With 192 miles of shoreline, which unlike Lake Powell, is mostly under private ownership, there would be opportunities for unlimited lakeside development. Promotors already have plans for Antelope Island. They see it as an ideal site for a theme park with high-rise hotels and condominiums.

Lake Wasatch is a chamber of commerce dream. Finally, the Great Salt Lake would be worth something.

What about the birds?

Mimi turns to me, her legs outstretched on the sands of Half-Moon Bay.

"How do you place a value on inspiration? How do you quantify the wildness of birds, when for the most part, they lead secret and anonymous lives?"

GREAT BLUE HERON

lake level: 4207.05'

A heron stands on the edge of the lake, solitary and serene. The wind shinnies up her back, raising a few feathers, but her focus remains steady. This is a bird who knows how to protect herself. She has weathered the changes well. Throughout the high water and now its retreat, the true blue heron has stayed home. Perhaps this is a generational stance, the legacy of her lineage.

I would like to believe she is reclusive at heart, in spite of the communal nesting of her species. I would like to wade along the edges with her, this great blue heron. She belongs to the meditation of water.

But then this is another paradox of mine—wanting to be a bird when I am human.

The gnostics teach me:

> For what is inside of you is what is outside of you and
> the one who fashions you on the outside is the one who
> shaped the inside of you. And what you see outside of
> you, you see inside of you, it is visible and it is your
> garment.

Refuge is not a place outside myself. Like the lone heron
who walks the shores of Great Salt Lake, I am adapting as
the world is adapting.

Mimi and I are on a Great Basin pilgrimage. It was
a trip I wanted to take while she still had her strength.

"Now tell me where we are going?" she asks.

"All I will tell you is that what Stonehenge is to England,
'Sun Tunnels' are to the Great Basin. At least, that's how I
choose to look at them."

We turn north off the interstate and eventually find our
way on a dirt road, which meanders through an endless sea
of sage. I explain how artist Nancy Holt spent three years,
from 1973 through 1976, creating "Sun Tunnels," how it is
a sculpture built on forty acres she bought in the West
Desert specifically as a site for the work.

Mimi puts on her glasses, opens an article on the sculpture
that I brought for her, and reads Nancy Holt's words out
loud:

> Sun Tunnels marks the yearly extreme positions of the
> sun on the horizon—the tunnels being aligned with the
> angles of the rising and the setting of the sun on the days
> of the solstices around June 21 and December 21. On
> those days the sun is centered through the tunnels, and
> is nearly centered for about ten days before and after the
> solstices.
>
> The four concrete tunnels are laid out on the desert

in an open X configuration eighty-six feet long on the diagonal. Each tunnel is eighteen feet long, and has an outside diameter of nine and a half feet and an inside diameter of eight feet, with a wall thickness of seven and a quarter inches.

Cut through the wall in the upper half of each tunnel are holes of four different sizes—seven, eight, nine, and ten inches in diameter. Each tunnel has a different configuration of holes corresponding to stars in four different constellations—Draco, Perseus, Columba, and Capricorn. The sizes of the holes vary relative to the magnitude of the stars to which they correspond. During the day, the sun shines through the holes, casting a changing pattern of pointed ellipses and circles of light on the bottom half of each tunnel. On nights when the moon is more than a quarter full, moonlight shines through the holes, casting its own paler pattern. The shapes and positions of the light cast differ from hour to hour, day to day, and season to season, relative to the positions of the sun and moon in the sky.

Each tunnel weighs twenty-two tons and rests on a buried concrete foundation. Due to the density, shape, and thickness of the concrete, the temperature is fifteen to twenty degrees cooler inside the tunnels in the heat of the day. There is also a considerable echo in the tunnels.

Mimi put down the article. "I can't wait to see them."

"I visited with Nancy Holt when I was in New York," I tell Mimi. "During our conversation, she talked about the process she personally underwent while conceiving them. She camped at the site for ten days and, at the time, wondered if she could stay in the desert that long. After a few days, she located a particular sound within the land and began to chant. This song became her connection to the Great Salt Lake desert. She told me she fluctuated from feeling very small to feeling very expansive. I remember her words, 'I became like the ebb and flow of light inside the tunnels.' "

"I understand that," Mimi says. "I remember going into my last surgery with two syllables in my mind, 'Ah, om,' 'Ah, om . . .' I closed my eyes and hummed those two words over and over until I was perfectly calm."

I stopped the car. "We're here."

Mimi looked out her window. "This is it? You mean these four pieces of conduit pipe? This looks like a job site of the Tempest Company!"

In Nancy Holt's "Sun Tunnels," the Great Basin landscape is framed within circles and we remember the shape of our planet, the shape of our eyes, our mouth in song and in prayer. These tunnels breathe as the ellipses expand and contract with the fickle light.

Smooth walls trick me into headstands, cartwheels, and somersaults. The sun hides and I want to say something—anything. The tunnels give import to my voice. It echoes. I laugh and chide and flirt with the gods until I find myself flat on my back with spots of sunlight covering my body—and I burst into tears, knowing it is only a matter of time until I am burned like paper beneath a magnifying glass. By morning, I will be left, frozen on the salt flats—forgotten forever were it not for my bones—bones that become whistles for the wind to blow through.

Mimi and I have not spoken for hours, each of us comfortable in our silences. A harrier hovers over the sage. Black, white, and gray. Male. I find a stash of feathers beneath the shadescale, I suspect horned lark. As I separate the brittle branches, sure enough, I find the foot with an extended hallax, lark for certain. A black beetle crosses the clay. One, two, three . . . seven, eight, nine mountain ranges are visible underneath this dome of sky.

I return to the east tunnel and fall asleep. When I awaken, I see Mimi standing in the center of the four "Sun Tunnels." She is turning slowly, looking outward in each direction.

ffffffff

SCREECH OWLS

fffffff

lake level: 4206.00'

Mimi passed away this morning at 5:10 A.M., June 27, 1989.

One week ago, she said to me, "You know, Terry, it's the strangest thing, I keep expecting to see an owl one morning."

"Have you ever seen an owl here?" I asked, looking out her bedroom window through the trees.

"No," she said.

"Have you ever heard one?"

"No, but I just keep thinking that one morning I will wake up to see an owl."

Four days later, I was lying next to her. We were talking. I took hold of her broad, square hand.

"Mimi, when you die, if there really is something beyond death will you send me a sign, so I will know you are fine?"

She looked at me with her eyes that always squinted when she smiled and laughed.

"It doesn't work. I asked my father the same thing and he never came back."

Jack sits quietly beside Mimi's body. A single candle burns on her dressing table. Reflected in the mirror, it appears as two.

Dad and Richard leave to call the family. I walk outside.

The sky is electric blue, the sycamore and horse chestnut trees are silhouetted in black. I walk down the porch, past the bedroom windows, to the privacy of the backyard. I think I hear the cooing of mourning doves above the lilacs. I look up to see them, but they are not doves at all.

They are owls. Two owls are circling each other on top of the telephone pole.

"Dance. Dance. Dance," I hear Mimi say.

I stand below them. One screech owl turns, faces me, then flies. The other owl turns. We stare. It lifts its wings over its head, flutters them, then disappears in the direction of the other.

> *Ah, not to be cut off,*
> *not through the slightest partition*
> *shut out from the law of the stars.*
> *The inner—what is it?*
> *if not intensified sky,*
> *hurled through with birds and deep*
> *with the winds of homecoming.*
> *—Rainer Maria Rilke*

Lying in my hammock at home, the wind rocks me back and forth. It is all that is left to comfort me.

Mimi and I shared a clandestine vision of things. I could afford to dream because she could interpret the story. We spoke through the shorthand of symbols: an egg, an owl. And most of what we shared was secret, much like the migrations of birds.

If I am to survive, I must let my secrets out like white doves held captive too long. I am a woman with wings.

With Mother I buried my innocence. With Mimi I will bury my haven.

Auden echoes from the open grave, "Our dreams of safety must disappear."

The Division of Water Resources has officially turned off the pumps. Great Salt Lake is on its own. The flood is over.

The Bear River Migratory Bird Refuge is able to breathe once again at lake level: 4206.00'.

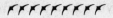

AVOCETS AND STILTS

ʄʄʄʄʄʄʄʄʄ

lake level: 4204.70'

The way to the Bird Refuge is clear for the first time in seven years. Great Salt Lake has retreated from sight, except for the faint line of silver on the horizon.

Refuge headquarters is unrecognizable. The buildings have been leveled. An old exhibit panel with a silhouette of a redhead flying over cattails stands akimbo among the wreckage. A partial title remains, reading simply, HISTORY—

Climbing over the rubble, spiders are everywhere. They are reinhabiting the Refuge. Their gossamer threads are binding it all together. Within minutes, I am draped with them. Even the avocets with their long, thin legs, sky blue, have silken strands trailing behind them.

The smell from the newly exposed land is ripe. Stilts walk on the cracked mud with skirts of brine flies around their red legs. Only a thin vein of water flows through the old canal, but volunteers have secured the banks. The U.S. Fish and Wildlife Service has promised $23 million toward the restoration of the Bear River Migratory Bird Refuge.

I turn. All at once, a thousand avocets take flight. More. Tens of thousands. A white and black flurry of birds circles me. The soft whistling of wings fills both time and space. I can no longer see the sky—above me, before me and behind me, avocets and stilts flock.

Oh, blessed wings.

In this moment, I realize how little I have hung on to for so long.

Brooke and I slip our red canoe into Half-Moon Bay. Great Salt Lake accepts us like a lover. We dip our wooden paddles into the icy waters and make strong, rapid strokes, north. The canoe powers gracefully ahead.

For two hours we paddle forward, toward the heart of the lake.

At the bow of the boat, I face the wind. Small waves take us up and down, up and down. The water, now bottle green, becomes a seesaw. We keep paddling.

The past seven years are with me. Mother and Mimi are present. The relationships continue—something I did not anticipate.

Flocks of pintails, mallards, and teals fly over us. There are other flocks behind them, undulating strands of birds like hieroglyphics that constantly rewrite themselves. Spring migration has begun.

We keep paddling. I have a turquoise and black shawl wrapped around me, protecting my face from the cold. This shawl is from Mexico, a gift to myself from the Day of the Dead.

I recall the impulse in me that said, "Go." I needed a ritual, a celebration to move me from death to life. I wore red for eight days—a simple cotton dress, drop-waisted and loose. I wanted no restrictions.

And when I entered the village of Tepotzlán, I bought flowers: gardenias, calla lilies, and lavender. But it was the marigolds that moved me. They were flames in the market-place. Villagers plant seeds in May to be harvested for this occasion. They call them *cempaxuchil,* the flower with one thousand blossoms.

In the *mercado,* there was a man purchasing masks of jaguar, frog, and deer. I watched him. He knew something. I bought a mask for myself, an owl made of papier-mâché.

The man left. I followed him through the market. He bought loaves of bread, chicken, molé, tomatoes, clumps of cilantro, basil, and thyme. In the plaza, he stopped and abruptly turned around. Our eyes met. I pretended to be buying incense.

"*¿Habla usted Inglés?*" I asked.

"*Sí,*" he said shifting his rucksack of food and masks to his other shoulder. (It turned out he was a North American who left the States in 1969. He had not been back since.)

"What should I know about *el Día de los Muertos?*"

He looked at me long and hard.

"What do you want from them?" he asked.

"From whom?" I responded.

"From your Dead."

I looked away.

"There is a small adobe up the hill. Look for a turquoise door. The Dead will be there—five o'clock tomorrow after-noon, the eve of *el Día de los Muertos.* If you are to find it . . . you will."

I found the turquoise door. A white gauze curtain was billowing from the doorway. As soon as I walked in, an old woman with a long gray braid running down her back led me out, behind the adobe, and baptized me in lime water.

Once inside, I sat down on one of the four white pews with a dozen or more villagers. It was a small white room. A woman knelt in front of a white altar, reciting prayers. Candles were burning. Thirteen candles. The shrine was smothered with white gladiolas. From one corner to the other, white crepe-paper flowers were strung between straws. The villagers prayed out loud with the kneeling woman.

I folded my hands across my lap and bowed my head. I was filled with gratitude for the graciousness of these people, that I could sit with them. A wave of emotion crested in me and broke. I wept silently for all I had lost. I reentered my own landscape of grief with perfect recall.

Songs were sung. More prayers were offered. And slowly my individual sorrow was absorbed into a sea of collective tears. We all wept.

Two women and a child, all dressed in white, sat in straight-backed chairs adjacent to the altar. In time, each one rose, trembling uncontrollably, sucking air through clenched teeth. They were in a quivering, hissing trance. I watched the Dead enter their bodies. They became taller, more robust, and confident. One by one, I listened to their stories. I watched their hands gesture the past as a mother spoke through her daughter, a sister spoke through her sister, and a mother spoke through her son.

After each account, the trembling and hissing returned, until the spirits slipped out through the storytellers' teeth and the peasants were returned to themselves. They collapsed, exhausted, back into the large white chairs.

Their stories were not so unlike my own. It was the reverberation of tone I recognized, like a piece of music you return to again and again that awakens the soul. The voices of my Dead came back to me.

Wearing my owl mask, I danced in the cobblestone streets. Bonfires lit every corner. Townsfolk circled them warming their hands. Tequila poured through the gutters. In one glance, I saw both lovers and murderers kissing and knifing each other against doors. Puppet shows were performed in the plaza as firecrackers exploded at our feet. Costumed children paraded through the village, carrying illuminated gourds as lanterns. All night long there is the relentless clamouring of bells, and the baying of dogs.

Carrying a lit candle, I entered the procession of masked individuals walking toward the cemetery. We followed the pathway of petals—marigold petals sprinkled so the Dead could follow.

The iron gates were open. Hundreds of candles were flickering as families left offerings on the graves of their kin: photographs, flowers, and food; calaveras—sugared skulls—among them. Men and women washed the blue-tiled tombs that rose from the ground like altars, while other relatives cut back the vines that obscured the names of their loved ones. There were no tears here.

A crescent moon rose above the mountains, a blood-red sickle.

"¿Por qué está aquí?" asked an old woman whose arms were wide with marigolds.

I looked up and stood. *"Mi madre está muerta."*

She points down. *"¿Aquí?"*

"No, no aquí"—not here. I try to explain in poor Spanish.

"She is buried back home, *Los Estados Unidos,* but this is a good place to remember her."

We both pause.

The woman motions me to another place in the cemetery. I follow her until she turns around. She slowly sweeps her hand across five or six graves.

"Mi familia," she says smiling. *"Mi esposo, mi madre y padre, mis niños."* Then her hand moves up as she recklessly waves to the sky. *"Muy bonito . . . este cielo arriba . . . con las nubes como las rosas . . . los Muertos están conmigos."* I translate her words. "Very beautiful—this sky above us . . . with clouds like roses . . . the Dead are among us."

She hands me a marigold.

"Gracias," I say to her. "This is the flower my mother planted each spring."

My mind returns to the lake. Our paddling has become a meditation. We are miles from shore. In sight are four blue islands: Stansbury Island on our right, Carrigan Island to our left, and straight ahead we can see Antelope Island and Fremont.

My hands are numb. We bring in our paddles and allow ourselves to float. Brooke pulls out a thermos from his pack and pours two cups of hot chocolate. I spread cream cheese over poppyseed bagels. We eat.

There is no place on earth I would rather be. Our red canoe becomes a piece of driftwood in the current. Swirls of brine shrimp eggs cloud the water. I dip my empty cup into the lake. It fills with them, tiny pink spherical eggs. They are a mystery to me. I return them. I lean into the bow of the canoe. Brooke leans into the stern. We are balanced in the lake. For what seems like hours, we float, simply staring at the sky, watching clouds, watching birds, and breathing.

A ring-billed gull flies over us, then another. I sit up and carefully take out a pouch from my pocket, untying the leather thong that has kept the delicate contents safe. Brooke sits up and leans forward. I shake petals into his hands and then into my own. Together we sprinkle marigold petals into Great Salt Lake.

My basin of tears.

My refuge.

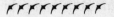

THE CLAN OF ONE=BREASTED WOMEN

Epilogue

I belong to a Clan of One-Breasted Women. My mother, my grandmothers, and six aunts have all had mastectomies. Seven are dead. The two who survive have just completed rounds of chemotherapy and radiation.

I've had my own problems: two biopsies for breast cancer and a small tumor between my ribs diagnosed as a "borderline malignancy."

This is my family history.

Most statistics tell us breast cancer is genetic, hereditary, with rising percentages attached to fatty diets, childlessness, or becoming pregnant after thirty. What they don't say is living in Utah may be the greatest hazard of all.

We are a Mormon family with roots in Utah since 1847. The "word of wisdom" in my family aligned us with good foods—no coffee, no tea, tobacco, or alcohol. For the most part, our women were finished having their babies by the time they were thirty. And only one faced breast cancer prior to 1960. Traditionally, as a group of people, Mormons have a low rate of cancer.

Is our family a cultural anomaly? The truth is, we didn't think about it. Those who did, usually the men, simply said, "bad genes." The women's attitude was stoic. Cancer was part of life. On February 16, 1971, the eve of my mother's surgery, I accidently picked up the telephone and overheard her ask my grandmother what she could expect.

"Diane, it is one of the most spiritual experiences you will ever encounter."

I quietly put down the receiver.

Two days later, my father took my brothers and me to the hospital to visit her. She met us in the lobby in a wheelchair. No bandages were visible. I'll never forget her radiance, the way she held herself in a purple velvet robe, and how she gathered us around her.

"Children, I am fine. I want you to know I felt the arms of God around me."

We believed her. My father cried. Our mother, his wife, was thirty-eight years old.

A little over a year after Mother's death, Dad and I were having dinner together. He had just returned from St. George, where the Tempest Company was completing the gas lines that would service southern Utah. He spoke of his love for the country, the sandstoned landscape, bare-boned and beautiful. He had just finished hiking the Kolob trail in Zion National Park. We got caught up in reminiscing, recalling with fondness our walk up Angel's Landing on his fiftieth birthday and the years our family had vacationed there.

Over dessert, I shared a recurring dream of mine. I told my father that for years, as long as I could remember, I saw this flash of light in the night in the desert—that this image had so permeated my being that I could not venture south without seeing it again, on the horizon, illuminating buttes and mesas.

"You did see it," he said.

"Saw what?"

"The bomb. The cloud. We were driving home from Riverside, California. You were sitting on Diane's lap. She was pregnant. In fact, I remember the day, September 7, 1957. We had just gotten out of the Service. We were driving north, past Las Vegas. It was an hour or so before dawn, when this explosion went off. We not only heard it, but felt it. I thought the oil tanker in front of us had blown up. We pulled over and suddenly, rising from the desert floor, we saw it, clearly, this golden-stemmed cloud, the mushroom. The sky seemed to vibrate with an eerie pink glow. Within a few minutes, a light ash was raining on the car."

I stared at my father.

"I thought you knew that," he said. "It was a common occurrence in the fifties."

It was at this moment that I realized the deceit I had been living under. Children growing up in the American Southwest, drinking contaminated milk from contaminated cows, even from the contaminated breasts of their mothers, my mother—members, years later, of the Clan of One-Breasted Women.

It is a well-known story in the Desert West, "The Day We Bombed Utah," or more accurately, the years we bombed Utah: above ground atomic testing in Nevada took place from January 27, 1951 through July 11, 1962. Not only were the winds blowing north covering "low-use segments of the population" with fallout and leaving sheep dead in their tracks, but the climate was right. The United States of the 1950s was red, white, and blue. The Korean War was raging. McCarthyism was rampant. Ike was it, and the cold war was hot. If you were against nuclear testing, you were for a communist regime.

Much has been written about this "American nuclear tragedy." Public health was secondary to national security. The Atomic Energy Commissioner, Thomas Murray, said, "Gentlemen, we must not let anything interfere with this series of tests, nothing."

Again and again, the American public was told by its government, in spite of burns, blisters, and nausea, "It has been found that the tests may be conducted with adequate assurance of safety under conditions prevailing at the bombing reservations." Assuaging public fears was simply a matter of public relations. "Your best action," an Atomic Energy Commission booklet read, "is not to be worried about fallout." A news release typical of the times stated, "We find no basis for concluding that harm to any individual has resulted from radioactive fallout."

On August 30, 1979, during Jimmy Carter's presidency, a suit was filed, *Irene Allen v. The United States of America.* Mrs. Allen's case was the first on an alphabetical list of twenty-four test cases, representative of nearly twelve hundred plaintiffs seeking compensation from the United States government for cancers caused by nuclear testing in Nevada.

Irene Allen lived in Hurricane, Utah. She was the mother of five children and had been widowed twice. Her first husband, with their two oldest boys, had watched the tests from the roof of the local high school. He died of leukemia in 1956. Her second husband died of pancreatic cancer in 1978.

In a town meeting conducted by Utah Senator Orrin Hatch, shortly before the suit was filed, Mrs. Allen said, "I am not blaming the government, I want you to know that, Senator Hatch. But I thought if my testimony could help in any way so this wouldn't happen again to any of the generations coming up after us . . . I am happy to be here this day to bear testimony of this."

God-fearing people. This is just one story in an anthology of thousands.

On May 10, 1984, Judge Bruce S. Jenkins handed down his opinion. Ten of the plaintiffs were awarded damages. It was the first time a federal court had determined that nuclear tests had been the cause of cancers. For the remaining fourteen test cases, the proof of causation was not sufficient. In spite of the split decision, it was considered a landmark ruling. It was not to remain so for long.

In April 1987, the Tenth Circuit Court of Appeals overturned Judge Jenkins's ruling on the ground that the United States was protected from suit by the legal doctrine of sovereign immunity, a centuries-old idea from England in the days of absolute monarchs.

In January 1988, the Supreme Court refused to review the Appeals Court decision. To our court system it does not matter whether the United States government was irresponsible, whether it lied to its citizens, or even that citizens died from the fallout of nuclear testing. What matters is that our government is immune: "The King can do no wrong."

In Mormon culture, authority is respected, obedience is revered, and independent thinking is not. I was taught as a young girl not to "make waves" or "rock the boat."

"Just let it go," Mother would say. "You know how you feel, that's what counts."

For many years, I have done just that—listened, observed, and quietly formed my own opinions, in a culture that rarely asks questions because it has all the answers. But one by one, I have watched the women in my family die common, heroic deaths. We sat in waiting rooms hoping for good news, but always receiving the bad. I cared for them, bathed their scarred bodies, and kept their secrets. I watched beautiful women become bald as Cytoxan, cisplatin, and Adriamycin were injected into their veins. I held their foreheads as they vomited green-black bile, and I shot them with morphine when the pain became inhuman. In the end, I witnessed their last peaceful breaths, becoming a midwife to the rebirth of their souls.

The price of obedience has become too high.

The fear and inability to question authority that ultimately killed rural communities in Utah during atmospheric testing of atomic weapons is the same fear I saw in my mother's body. Sheep. Dead sheep. The evidence is buried.

I cannot prove that my mother, Diane Dixon Tempest, or my grandmothers, Lettie Romney Dixon and Kathryn Blackett Tempest, along with my aunts developed cancer from nuclear fallout in Utah. But I can't prove they didn't.

My father's memory was correct. The September blast we drove through in 1957 was part of Operation Plumbbob, one of the most intensive series of bomb tests to be initiated. The flash of light in the night in the desert, which I had always thought was a dream, developed into a family nightmare. It took fourteen years, from 1957 to 1971, for cancer to manifest in my mother—the same time, Howard L. Andrews, an authority in radioactive fallout at the National Institutes of Health, says radiation cancer requires to become evident. The more I learn about what it means to be a "downwinder," the more questions I drown in.

What I do know, however, is that as a Mormon woman of the fifth generation of Latter-day Saints, I must question everything, even if it means losing my faith, even if it means becoming a member of a border tribe among my own people. Tolerating blind obedience in the name of patriotism or religion ultimately takes our lives.

When the Atomic Energy Commission described the country north of the Nevada Test Site as "virtually uninhabited desert terrain," my family and the birds at Great Salt Lake were some of the "virtual uninhabitants."

One night, I dreamed women from all over the world circled a blazing fire in the desert. They spoke of change, how they hold the moon in their bellies and wax and wane with its phases. They mocked the presumption of even-tempered beings and made promises that they would never fear the witch inside themselves. The women danced wildly as sparks broke away from the flames and entered the night sky as stars.

And they sang a song given to them by Shoshone grand-mothers:

Ah ne nah, nah	Consider the rabbits
nin nah nah—	How gently they walk on the earth—
ah ne nah, nah	Consider the rabbits
nin nah nah—	How gently they walk on the earth—
Nyaga mutzi	We remember them
oh ne nay—	We can walk gently also—
Nyaga mutzi	We remember them
oh ne nay—	We can walk gently also—

The women danced and drummed and sang for weeks, preparing themselves for what was to come. They would reclaim the desert for the sake of their children, for the sake of the land.

A few miles downwind from the fire circle, bombs were being tested. Rabbits felt the tremors. Their soft leather pads on paws and feet recognized the shaking sands, while the roots of mesquite and sage were smoldering. Rocks were hot from the inside out and dust devils hummed unnaturally. And each time there was another nuclear test, ravens watched the desert heave. Stretch marks appeared. The land was losing its muscle.

The women couldn't bear it any longer. They were mothers. They had suffered labor pains but always under the promise of birth. The red hot pains beneath the desert promised death only, as each bomb became a stillborn. A contract had been made and broken between human beings and the land. A new contract was being drawn by the women, who understood the fate of the earth as their own.

Under the cover of darkness, ten women slipped under a barbed-wire fence and entered the contaminated country. They were trespassing. They walked toward the town of Mercury, in moonlight, taking their cues from coyote, kit fox, antelope squirrel, and quail. They moved quietly and deliberately through the maze of Joshua trees. When a hint of daylight appeared they rested, drinking tea and sharing their rations of food. The women closed their eyes. The time had come to protest with the heart, that to deny one's genealogy with the earth was to commit treason against one's soul.

At dawn, the women draped themselves in mylar, wrapping long streamers of silver plastic around their arms to blow in the breeze. They wore clear masks, that became the faces of humanity. And when they arrived at the edge of Mercury, they carried all the butterflies of a summer day in their wombs. They paused to allow their courage to settle.

The town that forbids pregnant women and children to enter because of radiation risks was asleep. The women moved through the streets as winged messengers, twirling around each other in slow motion, peeking inside homes and watching the easy sleep of men and women. They were astonished by such stillness and periodically would utter a shrill note or low cry just to verify life.

The residents finally awoke to these strange apparitions. Some simply stared. Others called authorities, and in time, the women were apprehended by wary soldiers dressed in desert fatigues. They were taken to a white, square building on the other edge of Mercury. When asked who they were and why they were there, the women replied, "We are mothers and we have come to reclaim the desert for our children."

The soldiers arrested them. As the ten women were blindfolded and handcuffed, they began singing:

> You can't forbid us everything
> You can't forbid us to think—
> You can't forbid our tears to flow
> And you can't stop the songs that we sing.

The women continued to sing louder and louder, until they heard the voices of their sisters moving across the mesa:

> Ah ne nah, nah
> nin nah nah—
> Ah ne nah, nah
> nin nah nah—
> Nyaga mutzi
> oh ne nay—
> Nyaga mutzi
> oh ne nay—

"Call for reinforcements," one soldier said.

"We have," interrupted one woman, "we have—and you have no idea of our numbers."

I crossed the line at the Nevada Test Site and was arrested with nine other Utahns for trespassing on military lands. They are still conducting nuclear tests in the desert. Ours was an act of civil disobedience. But as I walked toward the town of Mercury, it was more than a gesture of peace. It was a gesture on behalf of the Clan of One-Breasted Women.

As one officer cinched the handcuffs around my wrists, another frisked my body. She found a pen and a pad of paper tucked inside my left boot.

"And these?" she asked sternly.

"Weapons," I replied.

Our eyes met. I smiled. She pulled the leg of my trousers back over my boot.

"Step forward, please," she said as she took my arm.

We were booked under an afternoon sun and bused to Tonopah, Nevada. It was a two-hour ride. This was familiar country. The Joshua trees standing their ground had been named by my ancestors, who believed they looked like prophets pointing west to the Promised Land. These were the same trees that bloomed each spring, flowers appearing like white flames in the Mojave. And I recalled a full moon in May, when Mother and I had walked among them, flushing out mourning doves and owls.

The bus stopped short of town. We were released.

The officials thought it was a cruel joke to leave us stranded in the desert with no way to get home. What they didn't realize was that we were home, soul-centered and strong, women who recognized the sweet smell of sage as fuel for our spirits.

ACKNOWLEDGEMENTS

First and foremost, I must honor my father, John Henry Tempest, III. He is a proud and private man. I thank him for understanding and respecting my desire to tell this story. He read each draft, edited and discussed the scaffolding of ideas built around a tender, and often-times painful, chronology. I have relied on his courage and vulnerability in trying to tell the truth. *Refuge* has been a collaborative project including my brothers and sister-in-law: Stephen Dixon Tempest, Daniel Dixon Tempest, and William Henry Tempest, each one for different reasons; Steve for his gravity, Dan for his perceptions, and Hank for feeling it all; my sister-in-law, Ann Peterson Tempest, invited me to be at the birth of their third daughter, Diane Kathryn Tempest, on January 27, 1990. Her gift was my healing. She intuitively knew I needed to see life coming in.

I thank my nieces, Callie and Sara, for their sweet companionship.

My grandfathers, Jack Tempest and Sanky Dixon quietly hold our family together. Both men in their mid-eighties continue to teach us about adaptability. For their wisdom, for their joy, I am indebted.

Ruth and Richard Tempest, Bob, Lynne, Michael, Matthew, and David; Steve Earl and Elizabeth Hansen Tempest. We are one tribe. Diane and Don Dixon, Debbie and Skip McWhorter, Shelley and Lee Johnson, Cami and Scott Dixon, Sean and Kerry Dixon; we share my mother's blood.

Marion Blackett, Norinne Tempest, Bea Berg, Ann Williams, and Natalie McCullough are relatives who offered insight into family matters. Extended family members; Blacketts, Bullens, Romneys, and Dixons offered physical and spiritual support. I thank them all for their web of concern.

Rex and Rosemary Williams have been a constant source of love in my life. To them, my debt is great.

To these friends, I owe a garden of flowers: Martha Moench, Jan Dalebout, Nancy Roberts, Roz Newmark, Hal Cannon, Meg Brady, Joan and Ted Major, Jack Turner, Med Bennett, Jan and Joey Williams, Becky and Dave Thomas, Nan and Steve Hasler, Amy and Tom Williams, David Brewer, Mary Beth Raynes, Sue and Thayer Christensen, Wangari Waigwa-Stone, Jeff Giese, Margy and Chris Noble, Glen Lathrop, Bruce Hucko, June Pace, Lynn Berryhill, Jeffrey Montague, Annick Smith, Bill Kittredge, Pauline Weggeland, Emma Lou Thayne, Margo and Fred Sylvester, Shelley and Rich Fenton, Gene Hoopes, Sally Smith, Beth Sundstrom, Greta DeJong, Flo Krall, Gwen Webster, Melissa and Scott Wood, Rich Wandschneider, P. K. Price, Donna Land Maldonado, Darci Cummins, Ron Barness, Betsy Burton, Patrick DeFrietas, Chet Morris, Steve Wilcox, Sam Weller, Steve Ashley, Karma Armstrong, Tom Lyon, G. Barnes, Kim Stafford, Sharon and Bill Loya, Marilyn Ellingson, Steve Casimiro, Liz Montague, Story and Bill Resor, Jim Harrison, and Barry Lopez.

My neighbors, John and Anne Milliken offered food, friendship, and retreat. Anne was my editor across the fence whose daily inquiries about my mother moved the manuscript forward. Conversations over tea turned into paragraphs.

I want to acknowledge the generosity of Lorna Miller and Don Albrecht at the Crescent H Ranch in Wilson, Wyoming; Heather Burgess of the Ucross Foundation; Jane and Ken Slight at Pack Creek Ranch in Moab, Utah; and Deborah Meier in New York City. They offered places of solitude in which to write.

Don Hague and the staff at the Utah Museum of Natural History are a remarkable community of individuals. They have my love and most sincere regard. Mary Gesicki in her grace, is responsible for creating an atmosphere I could work in.

Many individuals provided invaluable information that contributed greatly to the body of the manuscript and my understanding of Great Salt Lake. To their research and writings, I am indebted.

Dr. William H. Behle laid the foundation for all studies of birds at Great Salt Lake. *The Birds of Great Salt Lake* (University of Utah Press, 1958) remains a classic. I have used his research and knowledge extensively. His friendship and passion for ornithology have inspired me—first as his student and, later, as an instructor at the Utah Museum of Natural History. My love is his. Margy Halpin's bright soul inspired wonderful encounters and discussions surrounding the birds of Bear River, snowy plovers in particular. I acknowledge her expertise in reviewing the checklist. Peter Paton of Utah State University along with Anne Wallace provided biological data on snowy plovers and white pelicans. Sally Jackson and John A. Kadlec's work, "Recent Flooding of Wetlands Around Great Salt Lake, Utah," from the Department of Fisheries and Wildlife in Logan, Utah, was key in my understanding this complex ecosystem. A. Lee Foote offered insight into wetland ecology and plants important to waterfowl. The Utah Division of Wildlife Resources has been supportive of my work through the years: Tim Provan, Don Paul, Joel Huener, Tom Aldrich, Susan Aune, and Brenda Schussman, in particular. Their research, pacific flyway reports, and companionship in the field have been very valuable. Jim Barnes and Clayton White of Brigham Young University have offered ecological perspectives that altered my own, regarding birds and place. Emmett A. Alford, also of Brigham Young University, contributed to my understanding of white-faced ibises, their nesting behavior in relationship to habitat. Fred Ryser's work, *Birds of the Great Basin* (University of Nevada Press, 1985) has been central. Ella Sorenson has been my guide through taxonomy, along with Eric Reichart, curator of birds and mammals at the University of Utah. "Utah Birds: A Revised Checklist" by William H. Behle, Ella D. Sorenson, and Clayton M. White, *Occasional Publication,* No. 4 (Utah Museum of Natural History, 1985) has been my bible.

In the field of anthropology, David Madsen has been a star. His sense of Great Basin archaeology has broadened any understanding of what it means to live in arid country. Kevin Jones has been a companion in my understanding of Fremont culture. Our days at Floating Island were a gift. I have relied on their research and findings outlined in "The Silver Island Expedition, 1988," University of Utah Anthropological Papers (in press). Liz Manion's "Partial Analysis of Lakeside Cave Fauna" delivered at the XXI Great Basin Anthropology Conference was also helpful. Jim Kirkman, at the Utah State Antiquities office, took me through the excavation material and explained the meticulous process of cataloging. His knowledge is magic. Larry Davis and Dee Dee O'Brien were guides and helpmates down south in Anasazi country. Ann Hanniball, curator of collections at the Utah Museum of Natural History, has been my anchor through the maze of information always offering human insight into scientific equations. To her, I am indebted.

In my quest to understand Great Salt Lake, its fluctuations and geomorphology, I must thank especially Genevieve Atwood, Don R. Mabey, and Donald R. Currey. Their Map 73, "Major Levels of Great Salt Lake and Lake Bonneville" produced by the Utah Geological and Mineral Survey; Department of Natural Resources, gave me my blueprint of study. Without them, I am afraid I would have been reduced to metaphor. Standing out in the Basin, listening to them describe the lake levels, made Lake Bonneville a tangible presence. I found myself standing underwater. I also acknowledge their predecessors, G. K. Gilbert and R. J. Spencer. Ted Arnow, from the U.S. Geological Survey, also played a substantial role in my understanding. I am indebted to his work on water-level and water-quality changes in Great Salt Lake from 1843 to 1985. Ron Ollis of the Utah Division of Water Resources was extremely generous in his explanations of the West Desert Pumping Project. I used his research and public information materials heavily. Gode Davis and Cliff Nielsen wrote provocatively about the rise of Great Salt Lake in *Utah Holiday* (March 1987). I must thank them for their fine work which took me further into the politics of place associated with the flooding. Former Salt Lake City mayor Ted Wilson gave me a day of stories in the chronology of the State Street flood. His wit, wisdom, and savvy of Utah politics inspired me. Mark Rosenfeld reminded me that brine shrimp and brine fly larvae are not the only inhabitants of Great Salt Lake. I appreciate his sharing knowledge of fish in the Great Basin. Frank DeCourten, museum curator, was the individual who walked me through each lake level of Lake Bonneville and painted pictures of the Ice Age so vivid that I could no longer hold the Pleistocene Epoch as an abstraction. Lake levels have been supplied by the Utah Division of Water Resources.

In the medical profession, my heart goes to Dr. Gary Smith. He literally carried Mother and our family through death. And he did it with honesty, dignity, and compassion. He is family. Gary Johnson and Krehl Smith walked alongside. To these men, I am most grateful. The nursing staff at the LDS Hospital on 8 East was a beautiful expression of care, in particular, Faye Harder and Rolene Thompson. These were the women that Mother could be honest with and confide in without having to protect family. Dirk Noyes, Vicki Macy, and William F. Reilly were the caretakers of Mimi. They never lied. Hal Bourne, Hank Duffy, Howie Garber, and Steve Prescott also offered medical assurance along the way.

Natalie Clausen, Carol Mercereau, Marlisa DeJong, and Ann Kreilkamp, along with Rachel Bassett, were my healers. Women of great spirit.

The Mormon community we are a part of also healed us. I wish to acknowledge members of the Monument Park 11th and 14th wards. Bishop Craig Carman and Bishop Frank Nelson, in particular. Elder Hugh Pinnock brought both prayer and humor into our home through friendship. Beth Lords, Darlene Nilson, Joan James, and Diane Tonneson provided daily rituals which Mother relied on. Each one of her friends can write their name in here. Aenona and LaMar Crocker shared common ground. As a family, we honor the life of their daughter, Tamra Crocker Pulfer. Neighbors extend the notion of family. We were fed by them. Thank you.

Leonard Arrington has taught me about my own people. His thorough and thoughtful research into the history of Mormonism conveyed in *Brigham Young: American Moses* (Knopf, 1984) and *The Mormon Experience,* coauthored with Davis Bitton (Knopf, 1979), served as a catalyst and source for my discussions of the United Order, Brigham Young, and the early plight of the Latter-day Saints. I am grateful for his integrity in telling our history straight. He is trustworthy. Insights into Joseph Smith were gleaned from Michael Quinn's book, *Early Mormonism and the Magic World View* (Signature Books, 1987). Dale Morgan's vision of Great Salt Lake and its history has served as a baseline commentary. *Great Salt Lake—A Scientific, Historical and Economic Overview,* edited by J. Wallace Gwynn, Ph.D. (Utah Geological and Mineral Survey, 1980), has been an essential text.

Nancy Holt, the creator of "Sun Tunnels," was generous enough to let me into her home in New York where we shared our love of the Great Basin. I am indebted to her sense of place and her gift of forty acres outside Lucin, Utah. Most of the information used in this book came from direct quotations used in *Artforum* (April, 1977). Out of respect for her privacy, I chose not to draw from our personal conversations, rather allowed them to feed my own understanding of her work. Katie Nelson, a friend and art critic, first took me to the "Sun Tunnels." Once again, she drew me into the unseen world.

Regarding the epilogue, "The Clan of One-Breasted Women," I wish to thank Nini Rich who accompanied me to the Nevada Test Site in 1988. The stunning narrative of Philip L. Fradkin in his book *Fallout* (University of Arizona Press, 1989), provided the factual background of the essay. John G. Fuller also contributed to my understanding of nuclear politics in his book *The Day We Bombed Utah* (New American Library, 1984). To both men, I owe thanks. The Shoshone women who I was fortunate enough to cross the line with gave me their song. Carole Gallagher pushed me through my own denial. Her interviews and photographs of radiation victims are eloquently portrayed in *American Ground Zero: The Secret Nuclear War in the West* (MIT Press, 1993). The quotations "a good place to throw used razor blades" and "low-use segment of the population" come from a public lecture Ms. Gallagher delivered at the University of Utah, March 1988, and find their sources in declassified AEC top-secret material which she uncovered. Senator Orrin Hatch and Congressman Wayne Owens from Utah have been fierce advocates of downwinders, passing a compensation bill in the fall of 1990. Bless them. Don Snow and Deb Clow, editors of *Northern Lights*, are responsible for the original essay. They are alchemists. Howard Berkes of National Public Radio and Karen Rathe of the *Seattle Times* took the message further. Charles F. Wilkinson provided astute comments and legal guidance on the various court cases. His encouragement to be bold moved me beyond fear.

Tenia Holland and Kara Edwards provided perspective on the

manuscript as they worked with me on nuts and bolts. Linda Raw-lins provided accurate Spanish translations in my discussion of the Day of the Dead.

I have had dear traveling companions who have walked repeat-edly with me through this country: Lyn Dalebout, Dru Weggeland Brewer, Christopher Merrill, Jeff Foott, Laura Simms, Sandy Lopez (who kept me in flowers), and Ann Zwinger, who is my mentor. Lynne Ann Tempest shared my grief. Doug Peacock never fled from conversations of death. He stayed with me. To these friends, I express my devotion.

My family in New York, to whom I owe my professional life, were unwavering in their belief and support. Laurie Graham Schieffelin through her friendship and editorial wisdom crafted the manuscript. Linda Asher stretched the ideas and encouraged preci-sion of language. Carl Brandt held the vision of *Refuge* when I became weary. He never lost faith. He gave me mine. I especially want to thank Dan Frank, my editor at Pantheon, for his lack of sentimentality in his insistence that I tell the right story. We have traveled far together.

Lastly, I wish to express my deepest gratitude to my husband, Brooke Williams, who is fearless and wise in his capacity to love. He is bedrock.

BIRDS
ASSOCIATED WITH
GREAT SALT LAKE

Great Salt Lake supports a rich diversity and abundance of breeding, migrating, and wintering birds. Rare but regular species are included in this list, which has been organized according to the phylogenetic order used in common field guides.

Common Loon *Gavia immer*
Pied-billed Grebe *Podilymbus podiceps*
Horned Grebe *Podiceps auritus*
Eared Grebe *Podiceps nigricollis*
Clark's Grebe *Aechmophorus clarkii*
Western Grebe *Aechmophorus occidentalis*
American White Pelican *Pelecanus erythrorhynchos*
Double-crested Cormorant *Phalacrocorax auritus*
American Bittern *Botaurus lentiginosus*
Least Bittern *Ixobrychus exilis*
Great Blue Heron *Ardea herodias*
Great Egret *Casmerodius albus*
Snowy Egret *Egretta thula*
Cattle Egret *Bubulcus ibis*

Green-backed Heron   *Butorides striatus*
Black-crowned Night Heron   *Nycticorax nycticorax*
White-faced Ibis   *Plegadis chihi*
Tundra Swan (Whistling Swan)   *Cygnus columbianus*
Trumpeter Swan   *Cygnus buccinator*
Greater White-fronted Goose   *Anser albifrons*
Snow Goose   *Chen caerulescens*
Ross's Goose   *Chen rossii*
Brant   *Branta bernicla*
Canada Goose   *Branta canadensis*
Green-winged Teal   *Anas crecca*
Mallard   *Anas platyrhynchos*
Northern Pintail   *Anas acuta*
Blue-winged Teal   *Anas discors*
Cinnamon Teal   *Anas cyanoptera*
Northern Shoveler   *Anas clypeata*
Gadwall   *Anas strepera*
American Wigeon   *Anas americana*
Canvasback   *Aythya valisineria*
Redhead   *Aythya americana*
Ring-necked Duck   *Aythya collaris*
Greater Scaup   *Aythya marila*
Lesser Scaup   *Aythya affinis*
Oldsquaw   *Clangula hyemalis*
Surf Scoter   *Melanitta perspicillata*
White-winged Scoter   *Melanitta fusca*
Common Goldeneye   *Bucephala clangula*
Barrow's Goldeneye   *Bucephala islandica*
Bufflehead   *Bucephala albeola*
Hooded Merganser   *Lophodytes cucullatus*
Common Merganser   *Mergus merganser*
Red-breasted Merganser   *Mergus serrator*
Ruddy Duck   *Oxyura jamaicensis*
Turkey Vulture   *Cathartes aura*
Osprey   *Pandion haliaetus*
Bald Eagle   *Haliaeetus leucocephalus*
Northern Harrier (Marsh Hawk)   *Circus cyaneus*
Sharp-shinned Hawk   *Accipiter striatus*
Cooper's Hawk   *Accipiter cooperii*

Northern Goshawk   *Accipiter gentilis*
Swainson's Hawk   *Buteo swainsoni*
Red-tailed Hawk   *Buteo jamaicensis*
Ferruginous Hawk   *Buteo regalis*
Rough-legged Hawk   *Buteo lagopus*
Golden Eagle   *Aquila chrysaetos*
American Kestrel   *Falco sparverius*
Merlin   *Falco columbarius*
Peregrine Falcon   *Falco peregrinus*
Prairie Falcon   *Falco mexicanus*
Chukar   *Alectoris chukar*
Ring-necked Pheasant   *Phasianus colchicus*
Sage Grouse   *Centrocercus urophasianus*
Virginia Rail   *Rallus limicola*
Sora   *Porzana carolina*
Common Moorhen   *Gallinula chloropus*
Sandhill Crane   *Grus canadensis*
Black-bellied Plover   *Pluvialis squatarola*
Lesser Golden Plover   *Pluvialis dominica*
Snowy Plover   *Charadrius alexandrinus*
Semipalmated Plover   *Charadrius semipalmatus*
Killdeer   *Charadrius vociferus*
Black-necked Stilt   *Himantopus mexicanus*
American Avocet   *Recurvirostra americana*
Greater Yellowlegs   *Tringa melanoleuca*
Lesser Yellowlegs   *Tringa flavipes*
Solitary Sandpiper   *Tringa solitaria*
Willet   *Catoptrophorus semipalmatus*
Spotted Sandpiper   *Actitis macularia*
Whimbrel   *Numenius phaeopus*
Long-billed Curlew   *Numenius americanus*
Marbled Godwit   *Limosa fedoa*
Red Knot   *Calidris canutus*
Sanderling   *Calidris alba*
Semipalmated Sandpiper   *Calidris pusilla*
Western Sandpiper   *Calidris mauri*
Least Sandpiper   *Calidris minutilla*
Baird's Sandpiper   *Calidris bairdii*
Pectoral Sandpiper   *Calidris melanotos*

Dunlin   *Calidris alpina*
Stilt Sandpiper   *Calidris himantopus*
Long-billed Dowitcher   *Limnodromus scolopaceus*
Common Snipe   *Gallinago gallinago*
Wilson's Phalarope   *Phalaropus tricolor*
Red-necked Phalarope   *Phalaropus lobatus*
Franklin's Gull   *Larus pipixcan*
Bonaparte's Gull   *Larus philadelphia*
Ring-billed Gull   *Larus delawarensis*
California Gull   *Larus californicus*
Herring Gull   *Larus argentatus*
Thayer's Gull   *Larus thayeri*
Glaucous Gull   *Larus hyperboreus*
Caspian Tern   *Sterna caspia*
Common Tern   *Sterna hirundo*
Forster's Tern   *Sterna forsteri*
Black Tern   *Chlidonias niger*
Rock Dove   *Columba livia*
Mourning Dove   *Zenaida macroura*
Common Barn Owl   *Tyto alba*
Western Screech Owl   *Otus kennicottii*
Great Horned Owl   *Bubo virginianus*
Burrowing Owl   *Athene cunicularia*
Long-eared Owl   *Asio otus*
Short-eared Owl   *Asio flammeus*
Common Nighthawk   *Chordeiles minor*
Common Poorwill   *Phalaenoptilus nuttallii*
Black-chinned Hummingbird   *Archilochus alexandri*
Broad-tailed Hummingbird   *Selasphorus platycercus*
Rufous Hummingbird   *Selasphorus rufus*
Belted Kingfisher   *Ceryle alcyon*
Downy Woodpecker   *Picoides pubescens*
Hairy Woodpecker   *Picoides villosus*
Northern Flicker   *Colaptes auratus*
Western Wood Pewee   *Contopus sordidulus*
Willow Flycatcher   *Empidonax traillii*
Hammond's Flycatcher   *Empidonax hammondii*
Dusky Flycatcher   *Empidonax oberholseri*
Gray Flycatcher   *Empidonax wrightii*

Cordilleran Flycatcher   *Empidonax occidentalis*
Say's Phoebe   *Sayornis saya*
Western Kingbird   *Tyrannus verticalis*
Horned Lark   *Eremophila alpestris*
Tree Swallow   *Tachycineta bicolor*
Violet-green Swallow   *Tachycineta thalassina*
Northern Rough-winged Swallow   *Stelgidopteryx serripennis*
Bank Swallow   *Riparia riparia*
Cliff Swallow   *Hirundo pyrrhonota*
Barn Swallow   *Hirundo rustica*
Scrub Jay   *Aphelocoma coerulescens*
Black-billed Magpie   *Pica pica*
Common Raven   *Corvus corax*
Black-capped Chickadee   *Parus atricapillus*
Red-breasted Nuthatch   *Sitta canadensis*
Brown Creeper   *Certhia americana*
Rock Wren   *Salpinctes obsoletus*
House Wren   *Troglodytes aedon*
Marsh Wren   *Cistothorus palustris*
Golden-crowned Kinglet   *Regulus satrapa*
Ruby-crowned Kinglet   *Regulus calendula*
Mountain Bluebird   *Sialia currucoides*
Townsend's Solitaire   *Myadestes townsendi*
Hermit Thrush   *Catharus guttatus*
American Robin   *Turdus migratorius*
Gray Catbird   *Dumetella carolinensis*
Northern Mockingbird   *Mimus polyglottos*
Sage Thrasher   *Oreoscoptes montanus*
American Pipit   *Anthus rubescens*
Bohemian Waxwing   *Bombycilla garrulus*
Cedar Waxwing   *Bombycilla cedrorum*
Northern Shrike   *Lanius excubitor*
Loggerhead Shrike   *Lanius ludovicianus*
European Starling   *Sturnus vulgaris*
Solitary Vireo   *Vireo solitarius*
Warbling Vireo   *Vireo gilvus*
Orange-crowned Warbler   *Vermivora celata*
Virginia's Warbler   *Vermivora virginiae*
Yellow Warbler   *Dendroica petechia*

Yellow-rumped Warbler   *Dendroica coronata*
Black-throated Gray Warbler   *Dendroica nigrescens*
Townsend's Warbler   *Dendroica townsendi*
MacGillivray's Warbler   *Oporornis tolmiei*
Common Yellowthroat   *Geothylpis trichas*
Wilson's Warbler   *Wilsonia pusilla*
Yellow-breasted Chat   *Icteria virens*
Western Tanager   *Piranga ludoviciana*
Black-headed Grosbeak   *Pheucticus melanocephalu*⁻
Lazuli Bunting   *Passerina amoena*
Green-tailed Towhee   *Pipilo chlorurus*
Rufous-sided Towhee   *Pipilo erythrophthalmus*
American Tree Sparrow   *Spizella arborea*
Chipping Sparrow   *Spizella passerina*
Brewer's Sparrow   *Spizella breweri*
Vesper Sparrow   *Pooecetes gramineus*
Lark Sparrow   *Chondestes grammacus*
Sage Sparrow   *Amphispiza belli*
Savannah Sparrow   *Passerculus sandwichensis*
Grasshopper Sparrow   *Ammodramus savannarum*
Song Sparrow   *Melospiza melodia*
Lincoln's Sparrow   *Melospiza lincolnii*
White-crowned Sparrow   *Zonotrichia leucophrys*
Dark-eyed Junco   *Junco hyemalis*
Red-winged Blackbird   *Agelaius phoeniceus*
Western Meadowlark   *Sturnella neglecta*
Yellow-headed Blackbird   *Xanthocephalus xanthocephalus*
Brewer's Blackbird   *Euphagus cyanocephalus*
Brown-headed Cowbird   *Molothrus ater*
Northern Oriole   *Icterus galbula*
Cassin's Finch   *Carpodacus cassinii*
House Finch   *Carpodacus mexicanus*
Pine Siskin   *Carduelis pinus*
American Goldfinch   *Carduelis tristis*
Evening Grosbeak   *Coccothraustes vespertinus*
House Sparrow   *Passer domesticus*